Normal Electrophysiology, Substrates, and the Electrocardiographic Diagnosis of Cardiac Arrhythmias: Part I

Editors

LUIGI PADELETTI
GIUSEPPE BAGLIANI

CARDIAC ELECTROPHYSIOLOGY CLINICS

www.cardiacEP.theclinics.com

Consulting Editors
RANJAN K. THAKUR
ANDREA NATALE

September 2017 • Volume 9 • Number 3

ELSEVIER

1600 John F. Kennedy Boulevard • Suite 1800 • Philadelphia, Pennsylvania, 19103-2899

http://www.theclinics.com

CARDIAC ELECTROPHYSIOLOGY CLINICS Volume 9, Number 3
September 2017 ISSN 1877-9182, ISBN-13: 978-0-323-54544-0

Editor: Stacy Eastman
Developmental Editor: Donald Mumford

Cardiac Electrophysiology Clinics (ISSN 1877-9182) is published quarterly by Elsevier Inc., 360 Park Avenue South, New York, NY 10010-1710. Months of issue are March, June, September, and December. Subscription prices are $215.00 per year for US individuals, $331.00 per year for US institutions, $236.00 per year for Canadian individuals, $373.00 per year for Canadian institutions, $299.00 per year for international individuals, $399.00 per year for international institutions and $100.00 per year for US, Canadian and international students/residents. To receive student/resident rate, orders must be accompanied by name of affilliated institution, date of term, and the signature of program/residency coordinator on institution letterhead. Orders will be billed at individual rate until proof of status is received. Foreign air speed delivery is included in all Clinics subscription prices. All prices are subject to change without notice. **POSTMASTER:** Send address changes to Cardiac Electrophysiology Clinics, Elsevier Health Sciences Division, Subscription Customer Service, 3251 Riverport Lane, Maryland Heights, MO 63043. **Customer Service: 1-800-654-2452 (US and Canada). From outside of the US and Canada, call 314-477-8871. Fax: 314-447-8029. E-mail: JournalsCustomerService-usa@elsevier.com (for print support); JournalsOnlineSupport-usa@elsevier.com (for online support).**

Reprints. For copies of 100 or more of articles in this publication, please contact the Commercial Reprints Department, Elsevier Inc., 360 Park Avenue South, New York, NY 10010-1710. Tel.: 212-633-3874; Fax: 212-633-3820; E-mail: reprints@elsevier.com.

Cardiac Electrophysiology Clinics is covered in *MEDLINE/PubMed (Index Medicus)*.

Contributors

CONSULTING EDITORS

RANJAN K. THAKUR, MD, MPH, MBA, FACC, FHRS
Professor of Medicine and Director, Arrhythmia Service, Thoracic and Cardiovascular Institute, Sparrow Health System, Michigan State University, Lansing, Michigan, USA

ANDREA NATALE, MD, FACC, FHRS, FESC
Department of Cardiology, Texas Cardiac Arrhythmia Institute, St. David's Medical Center, Department of Biomedical Engineering, Cockrell School of Engineering, Department of Internal Medicine, Dell Medical School, University of Texas, Austin, Texas, USA; Department of Cardiology, MetroHealth Medical Center, Case Western Reserve University School of Medicine, Cleveland, Ohio, USA; Atrial Fibrillation and Arrhythmia Center, California Pacific Medical Center, San Francisco, California, USA; Division of Cardiology, Stanford University, Stanford, California, USA; Interventional Electrophysiology, Scripps Clinic, La Jolla, California, USA

EDITORS

LUIGI PADELETTI, MD
Heart and Vessels Department, University of Florence, Florence, Italy; Cardiology Department, IRCCS Multimedica, Sesto San Giovanni, Italy

GIUSEPPE BAGLIANI, MD
Arrhythmology Clinic Unit, Cardiology Department, Foligno General Hospital, Foligno, Italy; Cardiovascular Diseases Department, University of Perugia, Perugia, Italy

AUTHORS

GIUSEPPE BAGLIANI, MD
Arrhythmology Clinic Unit, Cardiology Department, Foligno General Hospital, Foligno, Italy; Cardiovascular Diseases Department, University of Perugia, Perugia, Italy

GIUSEPPE BORIANI, MD
Cardiology Department, Modena University Hospital, University of Modena and Reggio Emilia, Modena, Italy

ROBERTO DE PONTI, MD, FHRS
Cardiology Department, University of Insubria, Varese, Italy

DOMENICO GIOVANNI DELLA ROCCA, MD
Department of Cardiovascular Medicine, University of Rome Tor Vergata, Rome, Italy; Texas Cardiac Arrhythmia Institute, St. David's Medical Center, Austin, Texas, USA

LUIGI DI BIASE, MD, PhD
Texas Cardiac Arrhythmia Institute, St. David's Medical Center, Department of Biomedical Engineering, University of Texas, Austin, Texas, USA; Montefiore Medical Center, Albert Einstein College of Medicine, Bronx, New York, USA; Department of Clinical and Experimental Medicine, University of Foggia, Foggia, Italy

CAROLA GIANNI, MD, PhD
Texas Cardiac Arrhythmia Institute, St. David's
Medical Center, Austin, Texas, USA

FABIO LEONELLI, MD
Cardiology Department, James A. Haley
Veterans' Hospital, University South Florida,
Tampa, Florida, USA

DONATELLA LIPPI, MPH
Professor, Department of Experimental and
Clinical Medicine, University of Florence,
Florence, Italy

EMANUELA T. LOCATI, MD, PhD
Electrophysiology Unit, Cardiology Division,
Cardiovascular Department, Niguarda General
Hospital, Milan, Italy

ANDREA NATALE, MD, FACC, FHRS, FESC
Department of Cardiology, Texas Cardiac
Arrhythmia Institute, St. David's Medical

Center, Department of Biomedical
Engineering, Cockrell School of Engineering,
Department of Internal Medicine, Dell Medical
School, University of Texas, Austin, Texas,
USA; Department of Cardiology, MetroHealth
Medical Center, Case Western Reserve
University School of Medicine, Cleveland,
Ohio, USA; Atrial Fibrillation and Arrhythmia
Center, California Pacific Medical Center, San
Francisco, California, USA; Division of
Cardiology, Stanford University, Stanford,
California, USA; Interventional
Electrophysiology, Scripps Clinic, La Jolla,
California, USA

LUIGI PADELETTI, MD
Heart and Vessels Department, University of
Florence, Florence, Italy; Cardiology
Department, IRCCS Multimedica, Sesto San
Giovanni, Italy

Contents

reentry. Its classification is based on the atrial chamber involved and the arrhythmia's anatomic path. Ablative procedures for atrial fibrillation have created several new reentrant tachycardias. Electrocardiography (ECG) identifies the site of origin of focal atrial tachycardias and the mechanism of these arrhythmias. ECG is fundamental in the diagnosis of atrial fibrillation and often allows understanding of its mechanism of origin and maintenance.

The atrioventricular junction is a pivotal component of the cardiac conduction system, a key electrical relay site between the atria and the ventricles. The sophisticated functions carried out by the atrioventricular junction are possible for the presence of a complex apparatus made of specialized anatomic structures, cells with specific ion-channel expression, a well-organized spatial distribution of intercellular junctions (connexins), cells with intrinsic automatism, and a rich autonomic innervation. This article reviews the main anatomic and electrophysiologic features of the atrioventricular junction, with a focus on cardiac preexcitation.

The atrioventricular junction has a central role in electrophysiology, responsible for reentrant and automatic forms of supraventricular tachycardia. During atrioventricular nodal reentry tachycardia, the circuit involves 2 electrophysiologically separate pathways located in the vicinity of the atrioventricular node. Atrioventricular reentry tachycardia is caused by the presence of an accessory pathway located almost anywhere along the atrioventricular groove; the macroreentrant circuit involves the atrioventricular node, the accessory pathway and necessarily portions of atria and ventricles. Junctional tachycardia is a rare form of nonparoxysmal supraventricular tachycardia, secondary to enhanced automaticity or triggered activity. By analyzing a 12-lead electrocardiogram during sinus rhythm and tachycardia, it is possible to accurately diagnose the specific type of supraventricular tachycardia.

The ventricular conduction system starts below the His bundle, where it bifurcates into the right and left bundle branches that taper out to the subendocardial Purkinje network, which activates the ventricular myocardium. This system is responsible for the synchronized and almost simultaneous activation of both ventricles. On the surface electrocardiogram, the ventricular conduction system lies in the terminal portion of the PR interval, whereas the QRS complex composed of the electrical currents originating from ventricular depolarization. This article reviews the main electroanatomic features of the ventricular conduction system and the effects of its delay on the QRS.

Wide QRS complex is present when the normal activation pattern is modified by various mechanisms and clinical conditions. Correct interpretation is crucial for appropriate decision making. When approaching an electrocardiogram (ECG) with wide complex tachycardia, one must differentiate between ventricular tachycardia and supraventricular tachycardia conducted with aberrancy. ECG criteria are used and algorithms developed to aid in differential diagnosis. They are based on finding ECG signs of ventriculoatrial dissociation and QRS morphologies inconsistent with classic bundle branch block. The conditions able to modify structurally the normal activation of the heart may alter spontaneous ventricular activation during supraventricular tachycardia, creating differential diagnosis problems.

The QT interval on surface electrocardiogram represents the sum of depolarization and repolarization processes of the ventricles. The ventricular recovery process, reflected by ST segment and T wave, mainly depends on the transmembrane outward transport of potassium ions to reestablish the endocellular electronegativity. Outward potassium channels represent a heterogeneous family of ionic carriers, whose global kinetics are modulated by heart rate and autonomic nervous activity. Several cardiac and noncardiac drugs and disease conditions, and several mutations of genes encoding ionic channels, generating distinct genetic channelopathies, may affect the ventricular repolarization, provoke QT interval prolongation and shortening, and increase the susceptibility to ventricular arrhythmias.

CARDIAC ELECTROPHYSIOLOGY CLINICS

Foreword
On the Shoulder of Giants

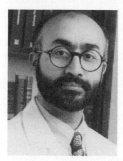
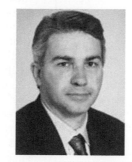

Ranjan K. Thakur, MD, MPH, MBA, FHRS Andrea Natale, MD, FACC, FHRS
Consulting Editors

The electrocardiogram is an essential part of a cardiovascular evaluation, following a detailed history and physical examination. This issue of *Cardiac Electrophysiology Clinics* is devoted to electrocardiography of arrhythmias.

Since the invention of the electrocardiogram in 1903, it has been utilized to learn much about cardiac arrhythmias as well as other cardiac abnormalities. Great scientists have contributed to our understanding of electrocardiography of cardiac arrhythmias. The editors of this issue were inspired by writings of Pick, Langendorf, Katz, and Schmaroth, and others during their formative years. As in other branches of science, it's a fitting tribute to say that present day arrhythmologists derive their contemporary understanding because they stand on the shoulders of giants from yesteryear.

The editors of this issue have taken a unique approach to discussing electrocardiography of arrhythmias. They first detail what can be learned about physiology, abnormality, and neural control from each wave and interval of the electrocardiogram and then build on that to discuss arrhythmias originating in each cardiac structure.

We congratulate Drs Padeletti and Bagliani and all the contributors for a unique approach. We hope the readers will enjoy reading and learning from their discussions.

Ranjan K. Thakur, MD, MPH, MBA, FHRS
Sparrow Thoracic and Cardiovascular Institute
Michigan State University
1200 East Michigan Avenue, Suite 580
Lansing, MI 48912, USA

Andrea Natale, MD, FACC, FHRS
Texas Cardiac Arrhythmia Institute
Center for Atrial Fibrillation at
St. David's Medical Center
1015 East 32nd Street, Suite 516
Austin, TX 78705, USA

E-mail addresses:
thakur@msu.edu (R.K. Thakur)
andrea.natale@stdavids.com (A. Natale)

Card Electrophysiol Clin 9 (2017) ix
http://dx.doi.org/10.1016/j.ccep.2017.07.002
1877-9182/17/© 2017 Published by Elsevier Inc.

Preface
Normal Electrophysiology, Substrates, and the Electrocardiographic Diagnosis of Cardiac Arrhythmias

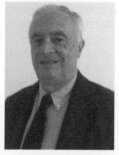 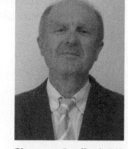

Luigi Padeletti, MD	Giuseppe Bagliani, MD

Editors

The purpose of this and the next issue of *Cardiac Electrophysiology Clinics* is to treat in depth and to review extensively any kind of cardiac arrhythmia defining the correct diagnostic approach on the surface electrocardiogram.

In the last decades, progress in basic research and in clinical electrophysiology has continuously increased our knowledge of the mechanisms underlying cardiac arrhythmias, furnishing evidence of previously undetected abnormalities of the formation and conduction of the cardiac impulse that help to make a correct electrocardiographic diagnosis of complex arrhythmias.

Basically, the focus of the issue is the surface electrocardiogram, with all the information we can obtain (from the cell electrophysiology to the neural control) in normal conditions and during rhythm disturbances. As a consequence, we followed a learning process starting from the description of the single electrocardiographic waves and intervals, which provides insight into

the physiologic and pathologic cause, the consequent morphologies, and the criteria of normality and abnormality. Successively, we developed the articles addressing the single arrhythmias originating in each cardiac structure, following a rationally based analytic approach to the accurate diagnosis of arrhythmias.

Our love for arrhythmology was aroused many years ago, when we were young fellows, by the papers and books of Katz, Pick, Langendorf, and Schamroth, Their methodology and rationality remain unreachable. Paraphrasing Isaac Newton, if next generations of arrhythmologists have seen further, it is by standing on the shoulders of these giants.

As the editors of this issue of *Cardiac Electrophysiology Clinics*, we would like to express our gratitude to the coauthors of the individual articles for their dedication to the production of these two issues. The donation of their expertise, time, and effort was essential. This issue also would not

Card Electrophysiol Clin 9 (2017) xi–xii
http://dx.doi.org/10.1016/j.ccep.2017.07.001
1877-9182/17/© 2017 Published by Elsevier Inc.

have been possible without the dedicated assistance of Donald Mumford. The support and encouragement of Ranjan Thakur and Andrea Natale were also essential.

Luigi Padeletti, MD
Heart and Vessels Department
University of Florence
Largo Brambilla, 3
50134 Florence, Italy

IRCCS Multimedica
Cardiology Department
Via Milanese, 300
20099 Sesto San Giovanni, Italy

Giuseppe Bagliani, MD
Arrhythmology Unit
Cardiology Department
Foligno General Hospital
Via Massimo Arcamone
06034 Foligno (PG), Italy

Cardiovascular Diseases Department
University of Perugia
Piazza Menghini 1
06129 Perugia, Italy

E-mail addresses:
luigi.padeletti@unifi.it (L. Padeletti)
giuseppe.bagliani@tim.it (G. Bagliani)

Arrhythmias in the History: Lovesickness

Donatella Lippi, MPH

KEYWORDS

- Lovesickness • Heart disease • Psychiatric disorders • Humoral disorders

KEY POINTS

- Lovesickness has been attested to in medical literature since classical times, and may still have a place in current medicine in psychiatry.
- The clinical use of pulse started with Galen, in the second century AD, who used it as a tool to diagnose disease and suggest possible treatments.
- Starting from the Middle Ages, lovesickness started to become a common subject also from an artistic point of view.
- The painter Jan Steen probably used Lovesickness to make fun of medical praxis of his times.

CLASSICAL TIMES

Lovesickness has been defined as "the most common form of heart disease."[1]

Lovesickness has been termed a real disorder, with a specific cause, pathogenesis, and cure: it has been attested to in medical literature since classical times, and may still have a place in current medicine in the frame of psychiatry and humoral disorders.

Although in different cultures there is a general agreement on the symptoms, including fever, agitation, loss of appetite, headache, rapid breathing, and palpitations, the treatments vary greatly in the various cultural contexts, from herbal remedies, to the prescription of sexual intercourse, to magical preparations.

The diagnosis was based on the Hippocratic semeiotic, which included anamnesis, observation, palpation, and succussion, but, starting from the fourth century BC, another criterion was developed: the description of pulse.

The protagonist of the story is the Prince Antiochus I Soter (324–261 BC), son of Apama and Seleucus I Nicanor, a military leader of the army of Alexander the Great and, after Alexander's death, founder of the Seleucid dynasty and of a mighty kingdom that extended from Syria to the river Indus.

When Antiochus was very young, he fell in love with Stratonices, daughter of Demetrius Poliorcetes, his father's second wife.

Because of this unethical feeling, Antiochus got sick and he was healed after many years by Erasistratus, a famous physician of antiquity: Erasistratus has been identified with different historical personages, from the mathematician Leptine[2] to Philippus.[3]

Valerius Maximus[2] provided many details in his description: Antiochus fell in love with his stepmother (*infinito amore correptus*) and tried to hide this deep and immoral wound of his soul (*impium pectoris vulnus pia dissimulatione contegebat*).

The description of the disease is very detailed: the ailment attacked Antiochus body, and he was close to dying (*iacebat ipse in lectulo moribondo similis*).

The only possible treatment was the union with the woman he loved, and King Seleucus, who was anxious to save his son, had no hesitation and offered him his wife (*Qui carissimam sibi coniugem filio cedere non dubitabit*). Seleucus, at the same time, gave to his son his wife, his kingdom, and his power.

All the investigators[2,3] agree that Erasistratus made his diagnosis by touching the pulse of the sick Antiochus: as Erasistratus felt Antiochus' wrist, he realized that the prince's pulse quickened

Department of Experimental and Clinical Medicine, University of Florence, Largo Brambilla, 3, 50134 Florence, Italy
E-mail address: donatella.lippi@unifi.it

Card Electrophysiol Clin 9 (2017) 341–344
http://dx.doi.org/10.1016/j.ccep.2017.05.008
1877-9182/17/© 2017 Elsevier Inc. All rights reserved.

and he became flushed when his stepmother Stratonice entered the room.

The attempt to measure pulse rate had been investigated in the same period by Herophilus (third century BC), who tried to compare the pulsation of blood vessels to musical rhythm, using a water clock that contained a specified amount of water for the natural pulse beats of each age group.[4]

However, the clinical use of pulse started with Galen, in the second century AD, who paid particular attention to an individual's pulse, monitoring it for abnormalities and using it as a tool to diagnose disease and suggest possible treatments.

For instance, using this system, Galen had detected that the little child Cyrillus had lied, because the wrist had become warmer and the pulse rate had accelerated: the discovery that the pulse has many variations, each variation carrying diagnostic or prognostic significance, led many investigators to try to describe the different movements of the blood in the radial artery.[5]

A situation similar to Antiochus' story is related about the young Prince Perdica, many centuries later, also concerning a medical reappraisal of the importance of the pulse.

In an undetermined moment of the late Roman period, Prince Perdica unintentionally became the victim of an incestuous love, which led him to death.

Perdica eventually killed himself, having suffered too much after having discovered that the woman he desperately loved was his mother.

The symptoms of Perdica's disease are consistent with those of Antiochus: insomnia, lack of appetite, hollowing of the eyes, anorexia, pallor, rapid pulse, jaundice.[6]

This kind of love, which developed into a real disease, was studied by the doctors, who suggested that this mental disorder should be classified as a variety of madness and a specific form of melancholy, because, in some cases, lycanthropy, flurries, stutter, and priapism may occur.

The Hippocratic-Galenic tradition had provided a basic humoral explanatory model: if love is unsatisfied, sorrow causes melancholy, caused by an excess of black bile.

MIDDLE AGES

In the Middle Ages, magic and temptations by demons were considered possible causes of lovesickness, but medical writings, based on the humoral approach to the disease, tried to explain it with the overheating of the vital spirit provoked by the object of desire, which, by inflaming the middle ventricle of the brain, the seat of the *virtus aestimativa* (faculty of estimation), caused dryness in the *virtus imaginativa* (faculty of imagination). The image of the beloved therefore became imprinted in the patient's memory, causing obsession.

Starting from the second half of the twelfth century, the term hereos came into use,[7] as a quasi-technical term to denote the disease of love.

The term, which was derived by a conflation of 2 distinct etymologic lines (love and hero), consistently denoted a pathologic version of love, shared by lovers whose sentiment was neither returned nor satisfied.

The first monograph in Western medicine on this subject was written by Arnaldo da Villanova (1240–1311): in his treatise *De amore heroico*, Arnaldo considered it not a disease (*morbus*), but a symptom (*accidens*), a peripheral presentation of a disease, derived from the modification of one of the 4 humors, which could easily degenerate into melancholy.[7]

During the Renaissance, lovesickness started to be considered not as a distinct disease but as a symptom, connected with a disorder, named in different ways: white fever, morbus virgineus, febris amatoria, characterized by pallor, amenorrhea, sadness, lack of appetite, palpitations. It was later named chlorosis, to underline a specific color of the skin, *ex albo ut plurimum virescente*.[8]

Lovesickness caused physical problems: erratic pulse, pallor, changes in appetite, and mood swings. The cure was usually marriage, which satisfied the needs of both the heart and the body.[9,10]

To this passion, which is able to provoke consumption, anorexia nervosa was also connected.[11]

MODERN ART

Lovesickness became a common subject in art during the seventeenth century, as in the pictures of the Dutch painter Jan Steen (1626–1679), who painted many scenes dedicated to this theme: the patient is always a young sick woman, suffering from lovesickness, and the doctor is shown while taking her pulse.[12]

At the heart of the matter there is usually a doctor visiting a patient. The doctor's clothing is outdated and looks more like theatrical costume from the *commedia dell'arte*. The physician seems out of date and out of touch with the condition of adolescent development.

The core subject of the painting is a weak young woman in a bed or chair, head resting on a cushion or table, while a doctor is taking her pulse. In the foreground there commonly are a ribbon dipped in urine, a blazing brazier, and a candle with chamber pot. The supposed illness is probably an unforeseen pregnancy, because the basin of coal with the burning thread was used by quack doctors in diagnosing pregnancy by reading the smoke, but, as an alternative, the unpleasant smell could cause a wandering uterus (*furor uterinus*) to return to its proper location. In this visual narrative, the diagnosis is clear to everyone except the doctor, because many details have an explicit sexual meaning. Lovesickness, known as minne-pijn (pain of the heart) or mine-koortz (fever of the heart) shared many of the symptoms of pregnancy, which was often part of the differential diagnosis.

In Steen's paintings, the doctor looks with apprehension at his patient as he takes her pulse. There are at least 2 main reasons for Jan Steen's interest in this subject. An apparent greater incidence of lovesickness in his times can be related either to a more skilled clinical eye, permitting increased detection, or to intention to make fun of doctors, who were so bad at seeking scientific evidence.

However, another reason is possible. In 1639 and 1643, Johan van Beverwijck (Beverovicius, 1594–1647), an established physician in the Dutch town of Dordrecht and already the author of popular medical works, published a treatise in which he described a particular disease that affected young women, in particular those who were widowed or childless in marriage.[13]

The cause is an intense sexual longing for a man. The signs and symptoms are protracted uterine cramps and dislocations (the furor uterinus). The patient is severely distracted, anxious, and depressed. On examination she is feverish, with an erratic pulse, and she feels hot and cold at the same time. The doctor suspects the diagnosis by observation only and/or by the exclusion of other conditions (such as pregnancy, female disorders, or intoxication), but the definite clue is the pulse test (pulsus amoris).

The ancient diagnostic technique of taking the pulse was long emblematic of the physician's ability to recognize otherwise hidden information about a sick person's condition.[14]

In Steen's times, practitioners could describe the regularity, frequency, strength, breadth, and depth of a pulse, using colorful expressions to name different conditions.

They could feel whether it was formicant or vermicular (antlike or wormlike) in motion, but they did not count.[5,15]

Although Galen argued that the arteries and heart contracted and dilated together, Harvey showed that the beat of the pulse coincided with the contraction of the heart, paving the way to the understanding of the mechanism of pulse rate.[5,16]

MODERN INSTRUMENTS

In Jan Steen's times, the Italian physician Santorius (1561–1636), from Padua, gave the first description of the circadian rhythm of cardiac frequency, inventing an instrument for the measurement and the comparison of the beats, the pulsilogium, or timepiece for counting pulses, which, according to his own statement, informed "in which period of the day and at which hour the patient's pulse changed in respect to the natural state."[17]

The seventeenth century's scientists had assimilated Galileo's lesson deeply, introducing quantitative methods into medicine and inventing many medical devices to measure the physiologic phenomena of human body.

Among them, Santorius is credited with inventing the earliest instrument to take the pulse rate, the pulsilogium.

Santorius was the first to use the physics of the pendulum to determine pulse rate, according to Galileo's observation that the frequency of the pendulum swing was inversely proportional to the square root of its length. The tool was a leaden bullet at the end of a linen or silk cord, and the oscillation on the pendulum was adjusted by changing the length of the cord, to match or synchronize with the pulse beat.[5]

The pulse rate corresponded with the position of a knot in the cord on a horizontal ruler, or the location of the hand on the dial.

The latter instrument had the cord wound around a drum, and, as the drum rotated to change the cord length, the hand moved around the dial.[5] In this way an evidence-based sphygmology was founded, scientifically clearing up many pathologic conditions. Lovesickness, which was considered a disease affecting the heart, could be taken as a model to investigate the interactions between pulse rate and progress of the disease, thus explaining the incidence of this condition in that historical period.

A Galenist in doctrine, Santorius applied the newly invented thermometer to medicine and also devised several other instruments, including the pulsilogium, which was also used by the Dutch physician and schoolmaster Isaac Beeckman (1588–1637), who was a great representative of the mechanical philosophy, and an expert technician.

According to Santorius, a pulse rate of "70 in degree" was considered normal.

The role of the physician in the use of the pulsilogium was pivotal, because he had to adjust the length of the pendulum until a periodic synchrony was achieved between pendulation and pulse.

The pulse rate was referred to in units of length, although it is rumored that one of those dial pulsilogiums took the form of a watch. Santorius observed and recorded the variations of pulse in the different hours of the day.

His example was followed by other scientists of the time. Some years later, Sir John Floyer[18]

(1649–1734) wrote *The Physician's Pulse-watch* (1707–1710), and he is credited with the invention of the first efficient instrument of precision to merit application in clinical practice.

Floyer set out to place sphygmology once more at the heart of medical practice, because he was sure that the pulse could reveal otherwise imperceptible information about the movement of the blood and other bodily fluids. It had been possible to "try pulses by the minute in common watches" since 1670, when the royal clockmaker, Daniel Quare, added a concentric minute hand to his watches: Floyer had used various clocks and watches, and had improved his accuracy by using a "Sea-Minute-Glass," which he had previously used to judge the length of time patients were immersed in a cold bath,[16] and later a portable pulse watch with an innovative second-hand was constructed for him by the skilled watchmaker, Samuel Watson.[19]

He then claimed to have discovered "a Rule whereby we may know the natural [and therefore healthy] Pulse, and the Excesses and Defects from that in Diseases." He asserted that the most basic way to discriminate between pulses was by recording the number of beats in a minute.[20]

From the collected data, Floyer argued that a healthy pulse was 70 to 75 beats per minute and that maladies were not only associated with but also produced by aberrant pulses and excessive or inadequate circulation, and suggested a therapy and regimen for reducing excessive, and raising deficient, pulses.

According to these observations, it is likely that Jan Steen depicted so many scenes of pulse-taking because this practice was commonly debated by scientists of the time and of his cultural context.

The more accurate ability to appreciate pulse variations had led the artistic eye to realize what the clinical eye had started to describe in the same years.

With the passing of time, lovesickness lost the original features, and the symptoms entered the realm of psychiatric disorders.

At the same time, doctors started to use more refined instruments to record pulse rate, paving the way for current sphygmology.[21]

REFERENCES

1. Dzaja N. Lovesickness: the most common form of heart disease. Univ West Ont Med J 2008; 78(1):66–9.

2. Kempf C, editor. Valerius maximus, factorum et dictorum meorabilium libri decem. Stuttgart (Germany): Teubner; 1966. V.7. ext. 1.

3. Poma R. Metamorfosi dell'hereos. Fonti medievali della psicofisiologia del mal d'amore in età moderna (XVI-XVII). Revue Des Littératures Européennes 2007;7:39–52.

4. Staden HV. Herophilus the art of medicine in early Alexandria. Cambridge (United Kingdom): Cambridge University Press; 1989.

5. Ghasemzadeh N, Zafari AM. A brief journey into the history of the arterial pulse. Cardiol Res Pract 2011; 2011:164832.

6. Zurli L, editor. Incerti auctoris, aegritudo perdicae. Leipzig (Germany): B. G. Teubner; 1987.

7. Lippi D, Verdi L, editors. Storia della magrezza. Corpo, mente, anoressia. Fidenza (Italy): Mattioli 1885; 2009.

8. Wells MA. Secret wound: love-melancholy and early modern romance. Stanford (CA): Stanford University Press; 2007.

9. Beecher DA, Ciavolella M. Jaques Ferrand. A treatise on lovesickness (1623) [transl. & comm.]. Syracuse (NY): Syracuse University Press; 1990.

10. Bynum B. Lovesickness. Lancet 2001;357:403.

11. Loudon IS. Chlorosis, anaemia, and anorexia nervosa. Br Med J 1980;281(6256):1669–75.

12. Oomen J, Gianotten WL. Lovesickness. Med Anthrop 2008;20(1):69–86.

13. van Beverwijck J, Von Haller A, van Esch H. 2: het tweede deel van den schat der gesontheyt. Waer in verhandelt wert, hoe ende op wat manier de verhaelde middelen: Tot Dordrecht: gedruckt by Hendrick van Esch, 1637.

14. Wallis F. Signs and senses: diagnosis and prognosis in early medieval pulse and urine texts. Soc Hist Med 2000;13:265–78.

15. Bedford DE. The ancient art of feeling the pulse. Br Heart J 1951;13:427–8.

16. Bylebyl JJ. Disputation and description in the renaissance pulse controversy. In: Wear A, French RK, Lonie IM, editors. The medical renaissance of the sixteenth century. Cambridge (United Kingdom): Cambridge University Press; 1985. p. 223–45.

17. Santorius S. Methodi vitandorum errorum omnium qui in arte medica contingunt. Geneva (Switzerland): Aubertum; 1631. p. 289.

18. Floyer SJ. The physician's pulse-watch; or, an essay to explain the old art of feeling the pulse and to improve it by the help of a pulse-watch, vol. I. London: S Smith and B Walford; 1707. p. 13.

19. Gibbs DD. The physician's pulse watch. Med Hist 1971;15:187–90.

20. Levett J, Agarwal G. The first man/machine interaction in medicine: the pulsilogium of Sanctorius. Med Instrum 1979;13(1):61–3.

21. Lippi D, Mascia G, Padeletti L. The pulsilogium and the diagnosis of love sickness. Hektoen Int 2014. Available at: http://hekint.org/tag/summer-2014/. Accessed June 1, 2017.

General Introduction, Classification, and Electrocardiographic Diagnosis of Cardiac Arrhythmias

Luigi Padeletti, MD[a,b], Giuseppe Bagliani, MD[c,d],*

KEYWORDS

- Cardiac electrophysiology • Normal heart rhythm • Electrocardiogram
- Cardiac arrhythmias diagnosis • Laddergram

KEY POINTS

- The electrocardiogram remains the primary instrument for detecting the electrical currents of the heart, both during normal and abnormal cardiac rhythm.
- Different mechanisms are at base of cardiac arrhythmias: impaired conduction, enhanced automaticity, or reentry.
- Electrocardiographic classifications concern the tendency to reduction or increase of the heart rate; well-defined sites of origin are the atria the atrioventricular junction and the ventricles.
- Particular forms of activation detectable both at atrial and ventricular levels are constituted by fibrillation and flutter.
- A rational method of analysis is the construction of the laddergram, a useful tool to make a rational diagnosis and to validate diagnostic hypotheses.

THE NORMAL CARDIAC RHYTHM

The complex apparatus of electrical activation of the heart is based on the presence of specific cardiac structures having the function of generating, conducting, and distributing the electrical signal to the contractile myocardium (**Fig. 1**). The function of generating the electric impulse is deputed to specific ionic channels located in particular cells whose activity is particularly pronounced in the sinus node (primary pacemaker); other cardiac structures, the secondary pacemakers, in "emergency" conditions can show pacemaker activity. The ability to create spontaneous depolarizations decreases as one moves away from the sinus node, and is lowest at the ventricular level.[1–3] The primary pacemaker receives important neurovegetative inputs, which regulate the frequency of depolarization, adapting it to the metabolic needs of the organism. The sinus impulse then spreads to the heart through the conduction system; the internodal tracts connect the sinus node to the atrioventricular node that constitutes the physiologic decelerator essential for optimum adjustment of the electromechanical delay between the atrial and ventricular conduction. Passed the atrioventricular node, the structures of the conduction system show high unidirectional conductive capabilities: the His bundle splits in the right and left branches, the latter with the division in 2

No relevant conflicts to disclose.
ª Heart and Vessels Department, University of Florence, Largo Brambilla, 3, 50134 Florence, Italy; ᵇ IRCCS Multimedica, Cardiology Department, Via Milanese, 300, 20099 Sesto San Giovanni, Italy; ᶜ Arrhythmology Unit, Cardiology Department, Foligno General Hospital, Via Massimo Arcamone, 06034 Foligno (PG), Italy; ᵈ Cardiovascular Diseases Department, University of Perugia, Piazza Menghini 1, 06129 Perugia, Italy
* Corresponding author. Via Centrale Umbra 17, 06038 Spello (PG), Italy.
E-mail address: giuseppe.bagliani@tim.it

Card Electrophysiol Clin 9 (2017) 345–363
http://dx.doi.org/10.1016/j.ccep.2017.05.009
1877-9182/17/© 2017 Elsevier Inc. All rights reserved.

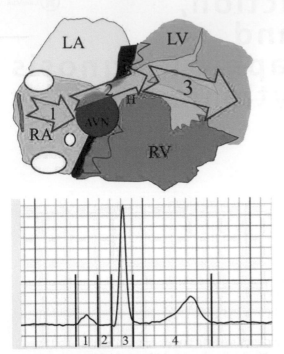

Fig. 1. The conduction system and the normal activation of the heart. 1 = P wave (atrial activation; 2 = PQ tract (junctional conduction); 1 + 2 = PQ interval; 3 = QRS complex (ventricular activation); 4 = ventricular repolarization; 3 + 4 = QT interval. AVN, atrioventricular node; AVN + His, atrioventricular junction; His, His, bundle; LA, left atrium, LV, left ventricle; RA, right atrium; RV, right ventricle.

fascicles (anterior and posterior); this trifascicular activation of the Purkinje system optimizes the contraction of the ventricles.

THE ELECTROCARDIOGRAPH AS A TOOL FOR DETECTION OF THE ELECTRICITY OF THE HEART: "CONDUCTION" AND "CONTRACTION" CURRENTS

In the heart, there are essentially 2 types of structures producing electrical currents: the conduction system and the contracting myocardium (atrial and ventricular).The cardiac conduction system, with sophisticated structures that depart from the upper part of the right atrium and arrive to the ventricles, produces currents of very low intensity, infinitesimally smaller than the ordinary atrial and ventricular myocardium.

The electrocardiogram (ECG) begins from the historical observations of the ability to detect the electrical currents transmitted from the heart to the body surface.[4,5] This is a process of conduction through which the currents are dispersed in a considerable manner, because it is possible to record from the body surface only about 1% of

the currents produced at the level of the heart. The conventional ECG is therefore a very weak system for the study of the currents of the heart; this difficulty that seems to be inherent to the method, remains unchanged in time, and does not seem to be overtaken by the various technological advancements, including digital acquisition.[6]

The surface ECG is, therefore, characterized by a series of methodologic difficulties that we can synthetically summarize in dispersion of electrical charges to the body surface, fusion of the currents produced by various structures, and morphology of the signals.

Dispersion of Electrical Charges to the Body Surface

The standard ECG is able to record only the electrical activity of the big myocardial masses, that is, the atria and the ventricles. Thus, the cardiac conduction system is absolutely not recordable from the body surface.

Fusion of the Currents Produced by Various Structures

The diffusion of electric charges of different structures leads to the merging of their currents with consequent formation of signals of summation of the original electrical phenomena: depolarization of the various parts of the atria will give the P wave, the "trifascicular" depolarization of the ventricles will generate the QRS, the repolarization of the ventricles will produce the QT. If the fusion phenomenon of the various currents produced by the heart is not problematic in the course of normal cardiac activation (because the signals themselves are clearly discernible from one another), during an arrhythmia, electrical events from different cardiac chambers change their temporal sequence, and overlap each other; this phenomenon represents a true interpretative difficulty in the diagnosis of cardiac arrhythmias (**Fig. 2**).

Morphology of the Signals

The slope of the recorded signals is an expression of the amount of current in the unit of time, and therefore will be low for the atria (rounded morphology with low amplitude) and high for the ventricles (the QRS components; **Fig. 3**). Considering the repolarization signals, they move in the opposite direction the same amount of electrical charges of the depolarization, but in a much longer time. This causes the almost complete disappearance of the signals of atrial repolarization and the formation of rounded shape signals of ventricular

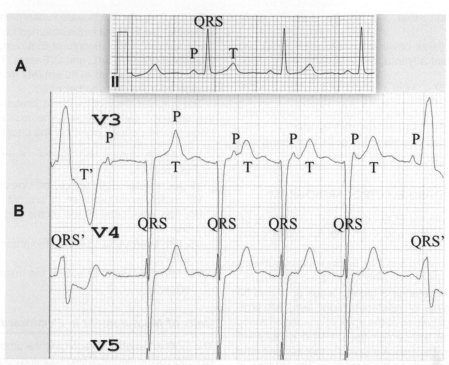

Fig. 2. The normal sinus rhythm (A) and a complex arrhythmia (B). The electrical activation of the heart during normal sinus rhythm shows a regular sequence of P-QRS-T waves. During the anomaly of cardiac rhythm 2 patterns of ventricular depolarization are evident (QRS and QRS') with corresponding different patterns of ventricular repolarization (T and T'). Atrial activity is regular and not clearly associated to ventricular depolarization (P waves are often superimposed to the ventricular repolarization).

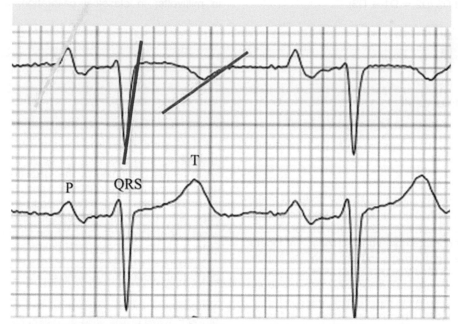

Fig. 3. The slope of the different signals of the heart depends on the currents produced by the single chambers: the slope is high for ventricular depolarization and slow for atrial depolarization. The repolarization of the ventricles produces smooth signals.

repolarization that constitutes the T wave complex.

Despite these obvious limitations the ECG has many evident advantages:

1. Extremely easy execution with great reproducibility;
2. Ease of identifying the signals that are constituted by amplitude/time curves; and
3. Maintained cultural value of ECG learning and experience during the years.

THE STANDARD ELECTROCARDIOGRAM

The conventional ECG consists of 12 leads, 6 on the frontal plane and 6 on the horizontal plane (**Fig. 4**).

On the frontal plane (**Fig. 5**), the initial hypothesis of the triangle of Eintoven[7] was based on the possibility of registering 3 bipolar leads (I, II, and III) from 3 points of reference (right arm, left arm, and left leg) placed at the apex of a triangle having the heart at the center: the D1 lead is obtained connecting the positive pole to the left arm and the negative pole to the right arm. The D2 lead is obtained by connecting the positive pole to the left leg and the negative pole to the right arm; the D3 lead is obtained by connecting the positive pole to the left leg and the negative pole to the left arm. The forces that come into play in 3 bipolar leads are governed by the law of Einthoven, according to which the D2 lead is equal to the sum of D2 and D3 (D2 = D1 + D3).

To the 3 bipolar leads were subsequently added 3 unipolar leads of the limbs obtained from each of the 3 apexes of the triangle of Eintoven; we have then obtained aVR, aVL, and aVF leads. The frontal plane is thus explored in its entirety from 6 leads staggered from one another of 30°.

The unipolar leads of the chest (precordial leads) are obtained by connecting the exploring electrode in well-defined points of the chest (**Fig. 6**):

V1: fourth intercostal space, right side of sternum.
V2: fourth intercostal space, left side of sternum.
V3: middle point between V2 and V4.
V4: fifth intercostal space on the mid clavicular line.
V5: fifth intercostal space on the anterior axillary artery.
V6: fifth intercostal space on the middle axillary artery.

Units of Measurement in Electrocardiography

The ECG is capable of recording the amplitude and direction of the electrical fields coming from the heart in relation with time. Therefore, the fundamental elements that must be taken into account when analyzing the morphology of a determined cardiac wave are the amplitude, duration, and polarity.

Unit of Amplitude of the Signals

The amplitude of the electrical signals is measured in millivolts; in classical calibration, a millivolt

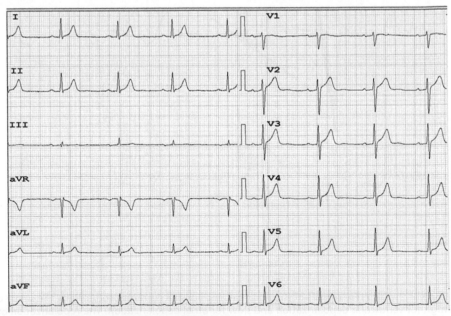

Fig. 4. A normal 12-lead electrocardiogram in an athlete.

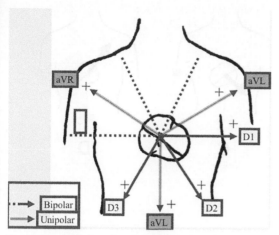

Fig. 5. The peripheral, unipolar, and bipolar leads.

corresponds with a signal amplitude of a centimeter (1 mV = 1 cm) (**Fig. 7**).

Unit of Time

The unit of time is shown in seconds or milliseconds; in classical calibration, the sliding speed of the paper is equal to 25 mm per second (25 mm/s; see **Fig. 7**).

Both of these units of measurement can be doubled or halved depending on your needs.

Calculation of the heart rate in a conventional electrocardiographic tracing: The conventional electrocardiographic tracing runs at the sliding speed of 25 mm per second (25 mm/s) and with amplification of 1 cm every millivolt. The electrocardiographic paper presents a more marked subdivision in the large square, whose side is equal to 0.5 cm (200 ms); a further subdivision is in smaller squares with side of 0.1 cm (40 ms). In an electrocardiographic tracing, standard heart rate can be

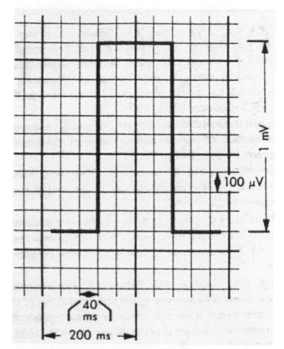

Fig. 7. The standard calibration of the electrographic signal: time on the x axis and Voltage on the y axis.

obtained by dividing the number 300 by the number of large squares that are contained between 2 QRS complexes.

Meaning and the Practical Usefulness of the Electrocardiogram Leads

The diagnostic specificity of each electrocardiographic lead must be known to browse to search for the maximum amount of information contained in it. It is usual to divide the ECG leads into groups that explore specific areas:

- Inferior leads: D2, D3, and aVF;
- Anterior leads: V1, V2, and V3; and
- Lateral leads: D1, aVL, V5, and V6.

The Cardiac Axis on the Frontal and Horizontal Plane

Cardiac axis on the horizontal plane
Fig. 8 shows how easy it is to determine a cardiac axis on the frontal plane by taking into consideration the polarity of the electrical event object of study, in 2 leads mutually perpendicular (D1 and aVF). We therefore have the following possibilities:

A. Normal electrical axis (between 0° and 90°)
    The normal electrical cardiac axis lies in the quadrant between 0 and 90°. Therefore, the global vector of QRS will be directed toward the positive pole of both leads

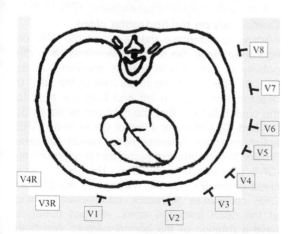

Fig. 6. The precordial leads.

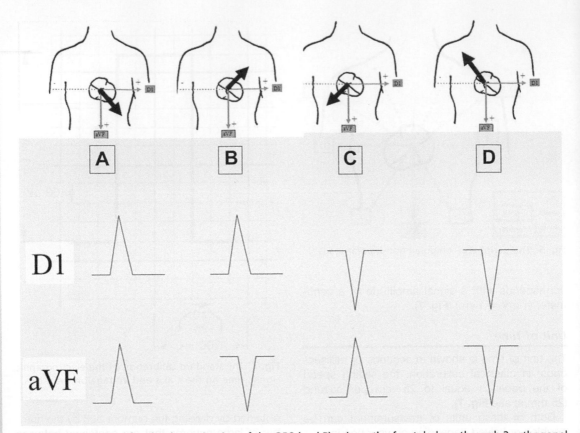

Fig. 8. Simple method for the determination of the QRS (and P) axis on the frontal plane through 2 orthogonal leads (D1 and aVF). (*A*) normal cardiac axis: it is directed towards the bottom and the left generating positive complexes in D1 and aVF; (*B*) left axial deviation: preserved positivity of D1, negativity of aVF; (*C*) right axial deviation: negativity of D1 and preserved positivity of aVF; (*D*) extreme axial deviation: this QRS axis, really not physiological, generates negative ventriculograms in D1 and aVF.

and the QRS will be positive in both leads D1 and aVF.

B. Left axis deviation (between 0° and −90°)
   A detour to the left of the electrical axis of the QRS occurs when the vector of ventricular activation is directed to the quadrant between 0 and -90°. The vector will be directed toward the negative pole of aVF and it will continue to remain facing toward the positive pole of D1. The QRS will be positive in D1 and negative in aVF.

C. Right axis deviation (between 90° and 180°)
   A detour to the right of the electrical axis of the heart occurs with a direct vector in the quadrant contained between 90° and 180°. The ventricular vector will be directed toward the negative pole of D1 and it will continue to remain facing toward the positive pole of aVF. The QRS will be negative in D1 and positive in aVF.

D. Indefinite electrical axis (between 180° and −90°)

A marked deviation of the cardiac axis both toward the right and toward the left lead the vector of ventricular activation to the upper right quadrant of the frontal plane. The QRS will be negative in D1 and in aVF.

Cardiac axis on the horizontal plane
Wishing to determine the vector of the QRS on horizontal plane, we must make reference to the polarity of the QRS in various precordial leads (**Fig. 9**). The normal electrical axis of the QRS is directed from right to left and from the front to the back.It follows that the right precordial leads (V1 and V2) will show a vector going away (QRS mainly negative), whereas the left precordial leads (V5 and V6) will record a vector that is approaching (QRS predominantly positive). The intermediate chest leads (V3 and V4) will register isodiphasic QRS complexes (transition complexes).Looking at the heart from the apex, we can therefore have a rotation of the normal cardiac axis both clockwise and counterclockwise.

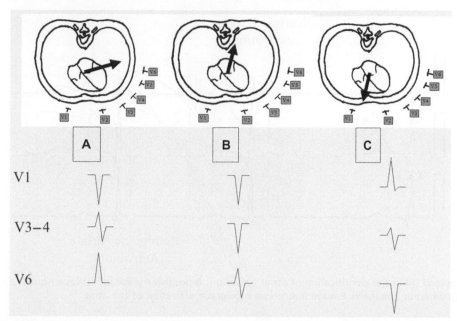

Fig. 9. Axial position of QRS on the longitudinal axis. (*A*) A normal cardiac axis is characterized by the negativity in V1, the positivity in V6 and transition complexes (RS pattern) in V3-V4; (*B*) Clock-wise rotation leads to a negativization also of V3 and V4 leads with transition complexes in V5-V6; (*C*) Counter clock-wise rotation: we observe ventriculograms that are mostly positive in V1, transition complexes in V3-V4 and negative in V6.

A clockwise rotation of the axis leads to the movement of the isodiphasic complexes toward the left precordial leads with negative complexes both in the right and intermediate precordial leads.In contrast, a counterclockwise rotation brings the isodiphasic complexes toward the right with negative complexes in both the intermediate and left precordial leads.

The D2 Lead and Atrial Activation as a Whole

The D2 lead, parallel to the front of atrial activation, is the optimal lead for analyzing the direction of atrial activation. In general, it should be kept in mind that, in the course of normal sinus rhythm, the P wave is positive in D2, implying a balanced activation of the 2 atria in a top-down direction. A negative P wave in the inferior leads generally indicates a retrograde atrial activation down-top of top-down type (**Fig. 10**), typical of the junctional and ventricular rhythms when they will be conducted back to the atria.

The V1 Lead and Ventricular Activation

The V1 lead is a unipolar lead particularly useful for the study of the ventricular activation. As will be explained elsewhere in this article, the lead V1 is a lead capable of recording the weak initial currents of the septal activation and is particularly useful for identifying the morphology of the so-

called wide QRS, that is, a type right bundle branch block if it is positive or type left bundle branch block if it is negative (**Fig. 11**).

HOW TO SEARCH FOR THE INDIVIDUAL POINTS TO DEFINE THE CRITERIA OF NORMALITY IN A STANDARD 12-LEAD ELECTROCARDIOGRAM

1. The isoelectric line is the horizontal line passing through the point of electrical silence, that is, after the end of the T wave and before the beginning of the P of the next cardiac cycle (see **Figs. 1** and **4**; **Fig. 12**). The isoelectric line defines in a certain sense the "zero point" of the ECG: each signal that is above the isoelectric line is defined as positive, whereas each signal that goes below it is defined as negative.
2. The P wave identifies the atrial activation; it is positive in D2.
3. The PQ interval identifies the duration of atrioventricular conduction as a whole and is measured from the beginning of the P wave to the beginning of the QRS.
4. The PQ tract is a limited tract between the end of the P wave to the onset of the QRS usually positioned on the isoelectric line, but in a way not to mistaken for it; the PQ tract contains information on atrial repolarization that usually

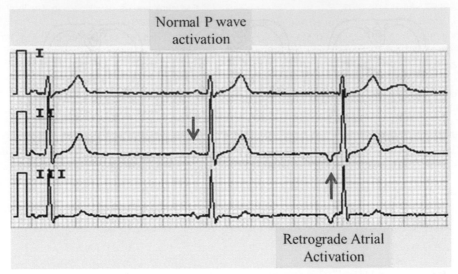

Fig. 10. The lead DII in the identification of atrial activation. A positive P wave identifies a normal atrial activation (sinus), whereas a negative P wave indicates a retrograde activation of the atria.

are very weak and, therefore, in normal condition, not modifying the isoelectricity of the PQ.

5. The QRS complex identifies the ventricular activation. To well-characterize the QRS, we should determine the duration and the electrical position on the frontal plane (QRS mainly positive in D1 and aVF) and horizontal plane (negative QRS in V1 and positive in V6, transition leads in V3-V4).

6. The J point is the fundamental point of passage between ventricular depolarization and repolarization. The J point is usually located on the

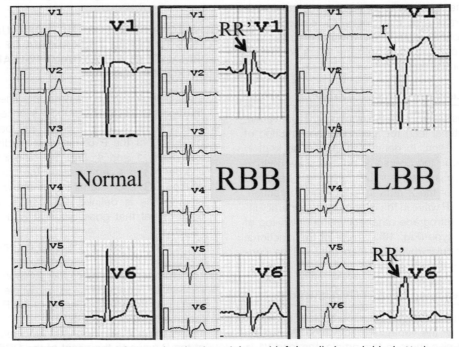

Fig. 11. Precordial leads in case of normal activation, right and left bundle branch block. Under normal conditions, there is a progressive positivation of the signals going from V1 to V6, with isodiphasic in V3. In case of right bundle branch (RBB) block, a pattern of double picking (R-R') is evident in V1 (and right precordial leads) instead in case of left bundle branch (LBB) block a similar pattern (R-R') is evident in V6 (and in left precordial leads).

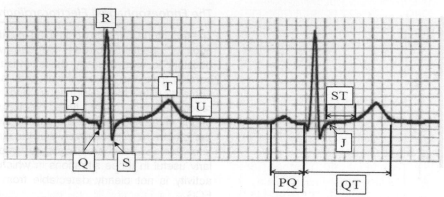

Fig. 12. Sequence of electrical activation of the heart as shown by the ECG. (1) P wave: atrial activation. (2) QRS complex: corresponds with the ventricular activation; it is made of 3 waves, of which 2 negative (Q and S) and a positive one (R). QRS ends in the J point, that is, where the ascending branch of S wave comes back isoelectric. (3) T wave: corresponds with the terminal phase of the ventricular repolarization. (4) U wave: not always well-evident. (5) PQ interval: it extends from the beginning of the P wave to the beginning of QRS; it comprises all the atrial activation, that one from the atrioventricular node and the His–Purkinje system. (6) ST tract: it extends from the J point to the beginning of the T wave, it is straight, horizontal, or slightly ascending and usually positioned on the isoelectric line. (7) QT interval: it comprises the time of ventricular depolarization and repolarization. Its duration is conventionally identified by the ventricular depolarization.

isoelectric line and it is important to identify if its location is either above or below it.

7. The QT interval usually identifies the duration of ventricular repolarization and can be calculated in absolute value or normalized to the ventricular rate with different formulas.

8. The ST segment is the first component of the ventricular repolarization and extends from the J point at the beginning of the T wave. It extends in a basically horizontal manner at the level of the isoelectric line.

9. The T wave is the terminal phase of ventricular repolarization; it is of monophasic morphology and usually with the same polarity of the QRS. In the composition of the T wave we can identify an ascending and a descending branch. Morphologic variations of the T wave may be attributed to ischemia, impaired concentration of blood electrolytes, and the effects of antiarrhythmic drugs and other drugs.

Analysis of the Basal Electrocardiogram

The analysis of the electrocardiographic tracing during sinus rhythm can be of particular importance in the identification of the substrates characteristically associated with particular arrhythmias. Thus, the anamnestic electrocardiographic confirmation of a ventricular preexcitation, a long QT, a previous myocardial infarction will orient respectively toward a supraventricular tachycardia, a torsade de pointes, or a ventricular tachyarrhythmia.

Of particular usefulness in the diagnosis of an arrhythmia with abnormal QRS can be the comparison of such QRS with the morphology of the ventricular complex during normal sinus rhythm or during an arrhythmia of known origin.

SYSTEMS FOR ALTERNATIVE AND COMPLEMENTARY ELECTROCARDIOGRAPHIC DETECTION

Some limitations of electrocardiography were considered insurmountable, especially because of the difficulty of recording structures that are far from the electrodes, although some alternative investigations can partially solve the problem.

The Endocavitary Electrocardiogram

Specific cardiac structures can be recorded using electrical catheters inserted in a venous access and whose electrodes are brought into direct contact with the cardiac structure object of study; the signal directly registered can be suitably amplified and filtered. The electrocardiographic recording of the bundle of His is the best expression of the endocavitary method; the electrocardiographic signal the bundle of His, a fundamental point of exploration of the atrioventricular junction, can be recorded easily with endocavitary technique as a quick signal positioned between the atrial and ventricular depolarization (**Fig. 13**).Reliable endocavitary signals can be also obtained from catheters of implanted systems (PACEMAKER and/or defibrillators), which therefore constitute an important diagnostic tool for the study of the heart rhythm.

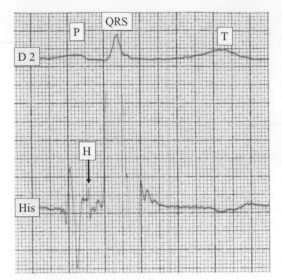

Fig. 13. His bundle recording. The potential of the His bundle (H), not evident on the electrocardiogram, can be recorded by using a catheter positioned inside the heart parallel to the same His bundle, amplifying and filtering the signal.

The Endoesophageal Electrocardiogram

The technique involves positioning into the esophagus of special electrodes through which it is possible to record easily the electrical currents coming from the left atrial wall, that is, in direct contact with the esophagus (**Fig. 14**); the recording made at this level, precisely because of the anatomic (and electrical) contiguity with the left atrium, will show very well the atrial activation. This special characteristic becomes particularly useful in those situations in which the atrial activity is not clearly detectable from a normal ECG.

By using recording apparatuses for electrophysiology, multiple points of the esophagus can be recorded simultaneously to characterize in sequence the left atrial activation. Also, the left atrial pacing is easily doable through the transesophageal lead; therefore, it is possible to use such an approach for diagnostic and therapeutic purposes.

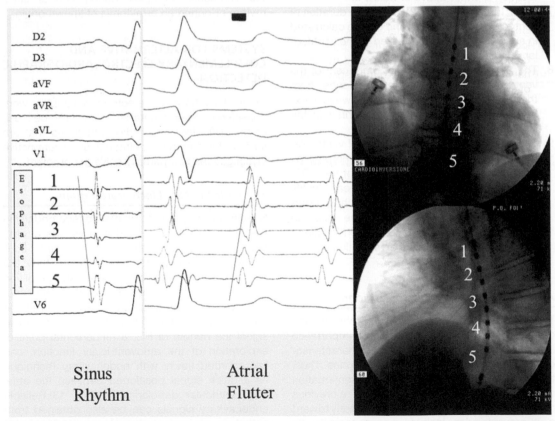

Fig. 14. Left atrial recording by multipolar esophageal lead. During sinus rhythm and counterclockwise atrial flutter. Two radiograms highlight—in posterior-anterior and lateral projection—the position of the left decapolar catheter, adjacent to the posterior wall of the left atrium that has a craniocaudal activation (*arrow from top to bottom*) in sinus rhythm, caudocranial (*arrow from bottom to top*) in case of atrial flutter.

Bipolar Chest Lead

Bipolar chest leads are used for dynamic registration of the ECG according to the method of Holter. Generally, 2 or 3 bipolar leads are used; if 3 leads are used, the electrodes are positioned in a manner similar to that of the orthogonal system X, Y, and Z.

Devices and Implanted Loop Recorders

A particular mode of obtaining an ECG is by the electrodes of a totally implantable recording systems. Nearly all pacemakers and implantable defibrillators have the ability to record electrocardiographic events. Implantable loop recorders are able to store an ECG signal automatically or externally activated by the patient.

THE GREAT CHALLENGE OF THE ELECTROCARDIOGRAPHY: IDENTIFYING THE ELECTROGENETIC MECHANISMS OF CARDIAC ARRHYTHMIAS
Bradycardias

The electrophysiologic mechanisms of bradycardia s are, within certain limits, immediately evident on the ECG: a reduced automaticity or a depression of the conductive system well explain the mechanisms of the bradycardias.

Automatic Arrhythmias

Cardiac arrhythmias by ectopic hyperautomatism frequently show a variation of the cycle, which is evident mainly as phenomena of warm up and cool down, respectively, at the beginning and at the end of the paroxysms (**Fig. 15**); the variation of the frequency of the heart chamber of origin is not so evident when episodes stabilize and are long lasting. There can be monomorphic and also polymorphic aspects of the activation chamber.

Reentrant Arrhythmias

Schematically, you need 2 conductive ways in electrical contiguity at their ends to produce a reentry; thus, a front of depolarization manages to take an anterograde direction and the other a retrograde direction for the reactivation of the starting point (**Fig. 16**). This conductive preference can only be realized if the 2 ways have different intrinsic electrophysiologic properties, that is, if they differ for conduction velocity and refractory period; in particular, some elements must be present for the realization and maintenance of a circuit of reentry:

- A slow pathway: characterized by a low conductivity and a short refractory period; and
- A fast pathway: characterized by a high conductivity and a long refractory period. Thus, it is not only a conduction difference that distinguishes the 2 pathways but, as is usually the case, also a difference of refractory period that should be shorter in the slow pathway: the reentry circuit is activated by a premature beat that can take the slow pathway in anterograde direction when the fast pathway is in its refractory period. The fast pathway is used for the retrograde conduction of the

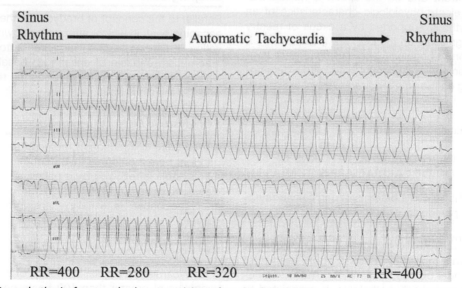

Fig. 15. An arrhythmia from exalted automaticity. After the first sinus beat, a ventricular tachycardia emerges with a characteristic trend: a variation of the cycle with the phenomena of the warming up (RR 400→280) and cooling down (280→320→400).

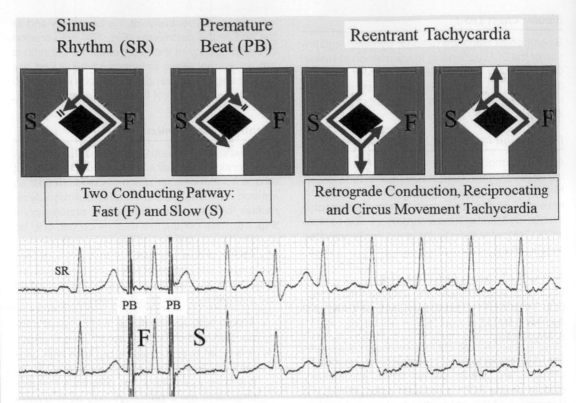

Fig. 16. Reentry arrhythmia (junctional reentry tachycardia). Two conductive ways (fast [F] and slow [S]) are necessary to produce a reentry. The 2 ways are in electrical contiguity at their ends. During sinus rhythm (SR) the front manages to reach the ventricles through the fast pathway but a premature beat (PB, induced in the electrophysiology laboratory) finds the fast pathway in the refractory period using the slow way to reach the ventricles (the PQ interval suddenly prolongs after the second PB). The F pathway is used for the retrograde conduction of the wavefront and so the circuit is maintained indefinitely.

wavefront and so the circuit is maintained. The electrophysiologic characteristics of an arrhythmia supported by a circuit of reentry recognizable on the ECG are therefore:

○ Abrupt beginning and end,
○ Constant cycle of the tachycardia depending on the time required to travel the circuit, and
○ Usually monomorphic activation of the chamber site of reentry.

ELECTROCARDIOGRAPHIC PATTERNS OF ACTIVATION OF CARDIAC ARRHYTHMIAS

Fig. 17 shows some patterns of particular arrhythmias morphologies.

Bradycardia

Bradycardia means a reduction of the heart rate, usually under 60 beats per minute. The phenomenon, not necessarily pathologic, is associated to the concept of a decreased electrical activation of a chamber.

Escaping Beat

Parallel to the concept of bradycardia there is the escaping beat, in which, after a slowdown of activation, a cardiac segment acquires autonomous automatism capable of ensuring a basal rhythm whose frequency is much lower as the rhythm is distal to the sinus node.

Extrasystolic Beat

A premature contraction of the heart that is independent from the normal rhythm of the heart. The extrasystole is followed by a pause, as the heart electrical system "resets" itself; the contraction after the pause is usually more forceful than normal.

Tachycardia

A tachycardia is a regular activation of the atria or ventricles of greater than 100 beats per minute. During a tachycardia, between a depolarization and the other, the isoelectric line is well-evident.

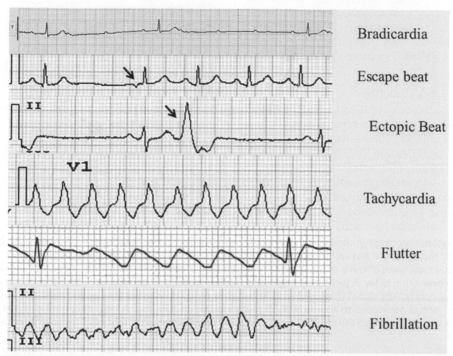

Right side labels for the ECG traces:
- Bradicardia
- Escape beat
- Ectopic Beat
- Tachycardia
- Flutter
- Fibrillation

Fig. 17. Some electrocardiographic presentation of cardiac arrhythmias. (1) Bradicardia: A reduction of the normal heart rate (under 60 bpm) is due to the a decreased electrical activation of a chamber (ventricular in this case). (2) Escaping beat after a relative reduction of the activation, a secondary pacemaker is able to give a cardiac segment acquires autonomous automatism (*arrow*). (3) Extrasystole: A premature contraction of the heart (ventricle in this case). The extrasystole is followed by a pause. (4) Tachycardia: This is an activation mode of a chamber (ventricular in this case) of the heart at a depolarization frequency clearly identifiable and reproducible from beat to beat, usually separated by an isoelectric line which is much less evident the higher the frequency is. (5) Flutter: This is a monomorphic form of tachycardic activation characterized by the alternation of phases of depolarization that obscure completely the repolarization and lead to the complete disappearance of the isoelectric line. (6) Fibrillation: electrical activity of chaotic depolarization with low or large fibrillation waves (atrial or ventricular), without an identifiable isoelectric line.

Flutter

Flutter is a monomorphic form of tachycardic activation characterized by continuous depolarization phases that obscure completely the repolarization and lead to the complete disappearance of the isoelectric line. Flutter-type activation is typical of atrial chambers even though the flutter term is used for some very rapid ventricular tachycardias in which the isoelectric line disappears.

Fibrillation

A fibrillation in the atrial or ventricular chambers is a very rapid and completely chaotic depolarization without any identifiable isoelectric line. The amplitude of the fibrillation waves can vary from very low to large. Although atrial fibrillation and ventricular fibrillation have the same electrocardiographic definition, their electrogenetic mechanisms and evolutions are completely different.

ANATOMIC AND ELECTROPHYSIOLOGIC CLASSIFICATION OF CARDIAC ARRHYTHMIAS

The possible locations of an arrhythmia have precise anatomic delimitation, clearly recognizable on the ECG.[8,9] From a point of view of functional electrical connections, the heart is divided into 3 parts: the atria, the atrioventricular junction, and the ventricles. This functional distinction is commonly represented in a laddergram (**Fig. 18**), which is a great tool of interpretative usefulness; the laddergram well-represents the syncytial functional units of the heart, namely, the atria, the ventricles, and the atrioventricular junction. The site of origin of the currents and electrocardiographic characteristics include the atria, atrioventricular junction, supraventricular and ventricular origin of the rhythm, and ventricles.

Atria

The atrial syncytial unit is constituted by the fusion of the left and right atrial mass whose electrical

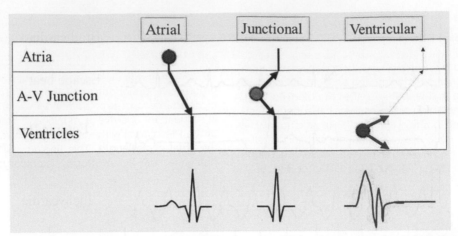

Fig. 18. Anatomic/electrophysiologic site of origin of an arrhythmia: the laddergram. The heart can be divided into 3 parts: the atria, the atrioventricular (A-V) junction, and the ventricles. An atrial origin is associated with an atrial activation wave (P wave or equivalent) followed by the ventricular activation; the 2 signals are separate by the A-V conduction delay. A junctional origin of a rhythm tends to depolarize the atrial and ventricular chambers simultaneously. Any signal that originates in the atria or in the atrioventricular junction is defined "supraventricular" and is associated to a narrow QRS (duration less of 120 ms). A beat originating in the ventricles generates a slowed-down activation which results in a wide beat (more than 120 ms) that can be retroconducted to the atria.

activity is usually dominated by the sinus node generating the normal sinus P wave, but the atria can also be abnormally activated as bradycardia, extrasystoles, tachycardia, flutter, and fibrillation.

Atrioventricular Junction

Anatomically, this site is the electrical junction between the atria and ventricles and is physiologically predisposed for bringing the atria to the ventricles; the atrioventricular junction can have conductive anomalies that may cause bradycardias, extrasystoles, and tachycardias. The atrioventricular junction does not have sufficient electrical mass to support autonomously a fibrillatory activity.

Supraventricular and Ventricular Origin of the Rhythm

Any rhythm that originates in the atria or in the atrioventricular junction is defined as supraventricular, and the limit of demarcation between the supraventricular and the ventricular zone is the bifurcation of the bundle of His. This limit is very important because the supraventricular QRS is usually narrow, differing from the ventricular one, which is wide.

Ventricles

The 2 ventricles represent a single syncytial unit activated by the specific conduction system. When the impulse originates in a point of the ventricular chambers, the electrical depolarization is able to activate the remaining ventricular mass both with a cell-to-cell conduction mechanism and by diffusion through the Purkinje system. The normal activation time of the ventricles and consequently the QRS duration is less than 120 ms. A QRS lasting 120 ms or more is defined as a wide QRS and represents an impaired activation of the ventricles, more often owing to a ventricular origin of the rhythm and less frequently to an intraventricular conduction delay of a supraventricular beat. Rarely, a wide QRS interval can also be due to a cardiac pacing or to a ventricular preexcitation.

During an arrhythmia, the ventricles may present anomalies of depolarization of all types, that is, bradycardias (especially conductive delays or branches delays), ectopias, tachycardias, flutter, or fibrillation.

ELECTROCARDIOGRAPHIC SUMMARY OF CARDIAC ARRHYTHMIAS

By previous electrophysiologic and anatomic assumptions, it seems to be obvious that an arrhythmia can occur on the ECG as bradycardia (heart rate <60 bpm), ectopic beats (single or coupled), or tachycardias (heart rate >100 bpm).

Bradycardias

Heart rate reduction below 60 beats per minute (or impaired conduction) owing to:

- Sinus bradycardia,
- Sinus arrest,

- Sinus atrial node block,
- First-degree atrioventricular block,
- Second-degree atrioventricular block,
- Third-degree atrioventricular block, and
- Bundle branch and fascicular blocks.

Extrasystoles

A premature depolarization of the heart; the site of origin can be located in the

- Atria,
- Junction, or
- Ventricles.

Tachycardia

Three or more consecutive beats at heart rate more of 100 beats per minute, which mechanism principally involves:

- The atria
    Sinus tachycardia
    Atrial tachycardia
    Atrial fibrillation
    Atrial flutter
- The atrioventricular junction
    Atrioventricular nodal reentrant tachycardia (common or slow/fast, not common or fast/slow, slow/slow)
    Atrioventricular reentrant tachycardia (orthodromic, antidromic, permanent junctional reentrant tachycardia, Mahaim fibers)
    Automatic junctional tachycardia
- The ventricles
    Monomorphic ventricular tachycardia (sustained and unsustained[a])
    Polymorphic ventricular tachycardia (sustained and unsustained[a])
    Torsade de pointes
    Ventricular flutter
    Ventricular fibrillation

THE LADDERGRAM: A RATIONAL APPROACH TO THE ELECTROCARDIOGRAPHY OF THE ARRHYTHMIAS

The analysis of the heart rhythm, be it normal or altered, requires the application of a simple, reliable method which allows to discover the electrogenetic mechanism of the arrhythmia itself, possibly representing the sequences of activation through the laddergram. From a practical point of view the, fundamental moments that should be followed to build a laddergram and then for the

electrocardiographic classification of an arrhythmia are (**Fig. 19**):

1. Identifying ventricular activity (QRS complex),
2. Identifying atrial activity (P waves or different atrial activation), and
3. Establishing relations between atrial and ventricular activity.

Mixing all the information obtained from the analysis of these points we have many useful data to diagnose an arrhythmia and only rarely will be necessary complex techniques (electrophysiologic studies) for the final diagnosis.

Analysis of the QRS Complexes

The electrical activity of the ventricles (QRS) is the largest electric component of an ECG and, therefore, it is usually of easy and immediate identification. Before you pass to any form of detailed analysis of the QRS you should realize if they are:

- Normofrequent, bradycardic, or tachycardic;
- Wide or narrow;
- Regular or irregular; and
- Monomorphic, polymorphic, or special forms of arrhythmia that is, fibrillation or torsade de pointes.

Once carried out, this simple initial assessment of the QRS complexes, other detailed elements will be taken into consideration.

QRS duration

From a methodologic point of view, the calculation of the duration of the QRS in the 12-lead ECG is the time elapsing between the early beginning of QRS and the end of the QRS in any surface lead. This implies that the beginning and the end of the QRS can be detected even in different leads so long as they are related to the same heartbeat.- From a descriptive standpoint, the QRS are generically defined as "narrow" or "wide" depending on which their duration is less or equal to or greater than 120 ms.

In general, a narrow QRS occurs for an origin of the impulse above the bifurcation of the bundle of His (supraventricular). A QRS that, in the course of an arrhythmia, is wide generally has a greater complexity of interpretation with respect to the narrow, because it is potentially an expression of a ventricular origin or a supraventricular origin with aberrancy of the intraventricular conduction (bundle branch block); more rarely, a

---

[a]Sustained/unsustained: an arrhythmia lasting more than or less than 30 seconds, or requiring or not requiring interventions for the arrhythmia resolution.

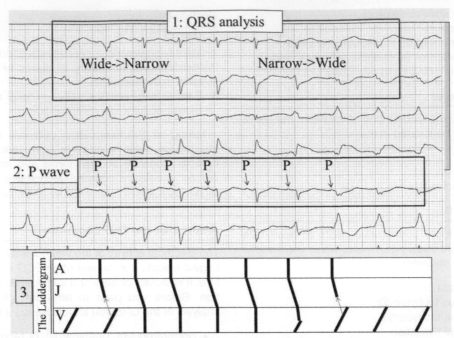

Fig. 19. The laddergram. Approach to the electrocardiogram of an arrhythmia by identify the QRS, the atrial activation, and the correlation between atria and ventricles (see text for further details). In this case, the first 3 and last 3 QRS are "wide QRS complexes." At the center, there is a series of 5 ventriculograms of normal morphology, each preceded by an evident P wave. The correlation of the events in the laddergram highlights the phenomenon of "ventricular capture" operated by the P wave. The final diagnosis is ventricular tachycardia and the transient ventricular capture is the "key" of the electrocardiogram.

wide QRS can be owing to a ventricular preexcitation or ventricular stimulation induced by a pacemaker.

QRS morphology

The criterion of duration is being able to identify the QRS as narrow or wide. Further data, especially useful for identifying the origin of the wide QRS, can be obtained from the morphologic analysis of the QRS. A wide QRS can present a monophasic, biphasic, or triphasic morphology (**Fig. 20**). Taking into consideration the morphology of the wide QRS in lead V1(see **Fig. 11**), it may be attributable to a pattern type right bundle branch block (positive in V1) or type left bundle branch block (negative in V1).

Rhythmicity of the QRS complexes

During normal sinus rhythm, RR intervals show very few variations, usually related to respiratory activity. A complete arrhythmicity of the QRSs is characteristically observed during atrial fibrillation. A sudden increase of the frequency of the heart is typical of the reentry arrhythmias of paroxysmal type, whereas arrhythmias based on hyperautomatism have a progressive increase in the frequency on the onset (warming up) and a

progressive reduction (cooling down) before the interruption.

Analysis of the P Waves

Identification of P waves

The identification of the electrical depolarization of the atria on the ECG is a fundamental point in the diagnosis of many arrhythmias. The P wave could be not evident in all leads and, therefore, it must be sought in detail in each of the 12 leads (usually D2 or V1). The P wave must be sought outside the QRS because the large vectorial forces of the QRS prevent a clear representation of small vector forces determined by the atrial activation; therefore, it does not seem to be methodologically correct to search for the P wave within the QRS to avoid that small deflections of the QRS are mistakenly exchanged for the P waves.

Very often during an arrhythmia, the P waves can fall immediately after the end of a QRS or inside a T wave, mimicking respectively bundle branch block or a T of abnormal morphology.In the case that P waves are not clearly evident, we have to consider one of the following situations:

1. The P waves are absent owing to lack of activity (sinus arrest or sinus atrial block);

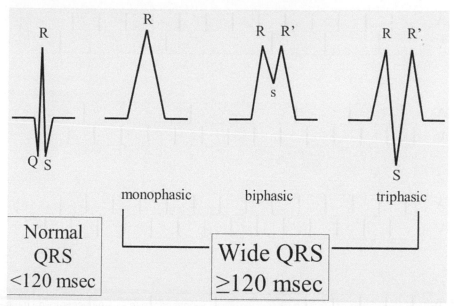

R   R   R   R'   R   R'

Q S

S   S

monophasic   biphasic   triphasic

| Normal QRS <120 msec | Wide QRS ≥120 msec |

Fig. 20. Pattern of normal and abnormal ventricular activation. One narrow and 3 wide ventricular activation (see text for further details).

2. The P waves are hidden inside other waves (especially the QRS or T); or
3. The P waves are replaced by other types of waves (fibrillation or flutter).

In cases of doubt when the surface ECG does not provide sufficient data for a clear identification, a valid alternative to the endocavity approach is constituted by the atrial recording by means of a transesophageal lead, positioned at the terminal portion of the esophagus where there is in direct contact with the posterior wall of the left atrium.

P wave morphology

The analysis of the axis of the vector of atrial activation is a useful element to identify the origin of the front of atrial activation and its subsequent direction of propagation (see Giuseppe Bagliani and colleagues, "P Wave and the Substrates of Arrhythmias Originating in the Atria," in this issue).

In the presence of normal sinus rhythm, the P wave is positive in the inferior leads (D2, D3, and aVf), implying a balanced activation of 2 atria in a top-down direction; a similar axis is presented by atrial rhythm originating in parasinusal position. A negative P wave in the inferior leads generally indicates a concentric atrial activation of a down-top type, typical of the junctional rhythms and of ventricular ones when they are conducted back to the atria. Eccentric atrial activations occur when an ectopic impulse originates in a portion of an atrium (left or right) and produces an impaired synchronism of the atria that leads to the development of particular atrial morphologies (see Giuseppe Bagliani

and colleagues, "P Wave and the Substrates of Arrhythmias Originating in the Atria," in this issue).

The Relationship Between P Waves and QRS Complexes

Once both QRS complexes and P waves are clearly identified, we must determine the relationship existing between the 2 events. This type of approach is particularly useful in the diagnosis of an arrhythmia. From a schematic point of view (**Fig. 21**) there are 4 possible cases.

A P/QRS ratio of greater than 1 indicates that the number of P waves is higher than that of the QRS complexes (eg, a ratio P/QRS = 4 indicates that every 4 P waves one is associated with a QRS). Generally, this pattern eventuality expresses a generic "filter action" of the atrioventricular node toward atrial tachycardias or for an impaired conduction in the atrioventricular node, making atrioventricular structures unable to propagate the normal atrial impulse to the ventricles. In any case a P/QRS ratio greater than 1 (commonly called second-degree atrioventricular block) indicates a supraventricular origin of the rhythm.

A P/QRS ratio of less than 1: the number of QRS is greater than that of P waves; this condition clearly indicates that the rhythm of the ventricles cannot be correlated in any way with the atrial activity as for a ventricular origin of the impulse (retroconducted to the atria with a particular conduction ratio).

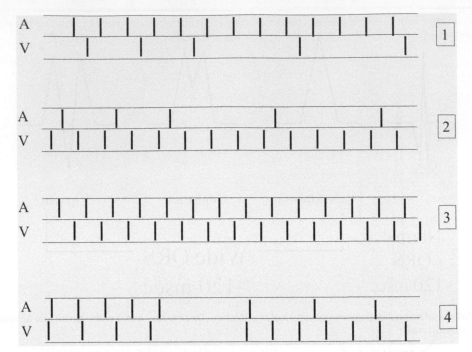

Fig. 21. The relationship between P waves and QRS complexes (see text for further details).

A P/QRS ratio of 1 indicates that every P wave is connected to a QRS. This condition, being observed in both supraventricular rhythm (each P manages to get to the ventricles) and ventricular rhythm (each QRS is stably retro-conducted to the atria). For this reason, a P/QRS ratio of 1 may not be used in the differential diagnosis between supraventricular and ventricular rhythm. When each P wave is associated to a QRS, other elements of extreme usefulness can be deducted from the analysis of the interval times between atrial and ventricular activity (the P-QRS interval and the QRS-P interval). Also, the pattern of activation of the atria (in particular the retrograde negative P in D2) is of particular usefulness.

The P and QRS are dissociated (atrioventricular dissociation): in this case, there is no association between atrial and ventricular activity and the 2 rhythms proceed autonomously. An atrioventricular dissociation can take place either for a conduction anomaly that prevents the atrial depolarizations to reach the ventricles or for a tachycardic rhythm originating in the ventricles with retrograde block of the conduction to the atria.

Effect of Vagal Maneuvers (and Drugs Equivalent) on the Atrioventricular Ratio

Vagal maneuvers, as well as medications that prolong the atrioventricular conduction up to the block (adenosine, verapamil, or digoxin), are commonly used in the diagnostic process of cardiac arrhythmias. During a tachycardia with a 1:1 atrioventricular ratio, vagal maneuvers may be particularly useful: the abrupt discontinuation of the arrhythmia means that the atrioventricular node is involved in the electrogenetic mechanism, but a lack of response does not help to determine any diagnosis. The reduction of the ventricular rate means a supraventricular tachycardia; differently, a constant ventricular rate associated to a reduction of the atria l rate means an origin of the rhythm at the ventricular level.

REFERENCES

1. Lewis T, Master AM. Observations upon conduction in the mammalian heart. A-V conduction. Heart 1925;12: 209–69.
2. Issa ZF, Miller JM, Zipes DP, editors. Clinical arrhythmology and electrophysiology: a companion to Braunwald's heart disease. 1st edition. Philadelphia: WB Saunders; 2009. p. 1–9.
3. Zipes DP, Jalife J, editors. Cardiac electrophysiology: from cell to bedside. 5th edition. St Louis (MO): WB Saunders; 2009.
4. Pérez-Riera AR, Marcus F. Evolution of the major discoveries in electrocardiology. J Electrocardiol 2015; 48(2):187.

5. Goldberger AL. Clinical electrocardiography: a simplified approach. 7th edition. St Louis (MO): Mosby; 2006.
6. Rosen M. The electrocardiogram 100 years later: electrical insights into molecular messages. Circulation 2002;106:2173–9.
7. Moukabary T. Willem Einthoven (1860–1927): father of electrocardiography. Cardiol J 2007;14:316–7.
8. Antzelevitch C, Burashnikov A. Overview of basic mechanisms of cardiac arrhythmia. Card Electrophysiol Clin 2011;3:23–45.
9. Jalife J, Delmar M, Anumonwo J, et al. Basic mechanisms of cardiac arrhythmias. Basic cardiac electrophysiology for the clinician. 2nd edition. Oxford: Wiley-Blackwell; 2009.

P Wave and the Substrates of Arrhythmias Originating in the Atria

 CrossMark

Giuseppe Bagliani, MD[a,b],*, Fabio Leonelli, MD[c], Luigi Padeletti, MD[d,e]

KEYWORDS

- Atrial sinus node • Atrial activation • Normal P wave • Ectopic P wave • Wandering pacemaker
- Paced P wave • Atrial arrhythmias

KEY POINTS

- Sinus node is a complex structure with automatic properties, capable of determining optimal cardiac rate and depolarizing the atria using a well-structured impulse conduction system.
- P wave analysis provides a wealth of information regarding automatic function, conduction, and global atrial activation during both normal and pathologic function.
- Specific structural anomalies are the substrate for re-entrant and focal atrial arrhythmias' mechanisms.
- Electrocardiographic analysis is an accurate diagnostic tool to define atrial flutter, atrial fibrillation, and atrial tachycardias.

INTRODUCTION

The systematic approach to the analysis of the P wave's normal and abnormal patterns and variations requires basic knowledge of the anatomic and functional ionic mechanisms of atrial activation.

The atria function as a conduit between the ventricles and venous and pulmonary circulation, contributing with active contraction to ventricular filling. To optimize contraction, atria need to generate an electrical impulse and disperse this activation to both chambers in a sequential fashion. To achieve this goal, the atria require a group of automatic cells and muscle fibers oriented to steer the depolarizing wavefront to obtain the most effective torsion-like contraction (**Fig. 1**). Devoid of a specialized conduction system, the atria direct the electrical wavefront by orienting its progression along the myocytes long axis. Conduction impedance is markedly decreased along the longitudinal axis compared with the transverse.[1]

It is well known that the primary pacemaker; that is, the one with the highest heart rate able to dominate all the secondary (accessory) pacemakers, is the sinoatrial node (SN). The SN is located at the junction between the lateral wall of the right atrium and the superior vena cava where the heart's conduction process takes place.[1,2] The atrial activation front propagates from the SN to the contiguous right atrium passing through a

No relevant conflicts to disclose.
[a] Arrhythmology Unit, Cardiology Department, Foligno General Hospital, Via Massimo Arcamone, 06034 Foligno (PG), Italy; [b] Cardiovascular Diseases Department, University of Perugia, Piazza Menghini 1, 06129 Perugia, Italy, [c] Cardiology Department James A. Haley Veterans' Hospital, University South Florida, 13000 Bruce B Down Boulevard, Tampa, FL 33612, USA; [d] Heart and Vessels Department, University of Florence, Largo Brambilla, 3, 50134 Florence, Italy; [e] IRCCS Multimedica, Cardiology Department, Via Milanese, 300, 20099 Sesto San Giovanni, Italy
* Corresponding author. Via Centrale Umbra 17, 06038 Spello (PG), Italy.
E-mail address: giuseppe.bagliani@tim.it

Card Electrophysiol Clin 9 (2017) 365–382
http://dx.doi.org/10.1016/j.ccep.2017.05.001
1877-9182/17/© 2017 Elsevier Inc. All rights reserved.

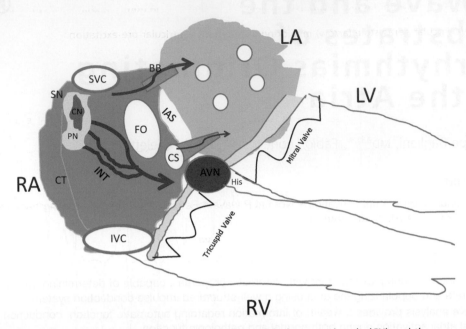

Fig. 1. The conduction system of the atria. Sinus node (SN), with the central node (CN) and the paranodal zone (PN). Atrioventricular node (AVN) and the internodal tract (INT). Interatrial conduction with the Bachmann Bundle (BB) and atrial fibers of coronary sinus (CS). CT, crista terminalis; FO, fossa ovalis; IAS, interatrial septum; LA, left atrium; LV, left ventricle; RA, right atrium; RV, right ventricle; SVC, superior vena cava.

well-organized structure constituted by the paranodal (PN) zone.

A well-organized trabecular bundle of atrial fibers guarantees the impulse propagation to the atrioventricular (AV) node via specialized pathways known as internodal tracts. Although it was once thought that the left atrial activation was a direct propagation of the activation front coming from the right atrium, the conduction between the 2 atria is ensured by the presence of particular structures located at the top and the bottom of the right atrium: the Bachmann bundle (BB) and the muscle tissue of the coronary sinus (CS), respectively. This interatrial conduction system determines the conduction mode and, consequently, the P wave morphology on electrocardiogram (ECG).

SINUS ATRIAL NODE

The SN is the structure in which electrical impulses are normally generated in the heart.

The elements that characterize the SN's function are the generation of the electrical impulse and its propagation to the surrounding atrial muscle. The electrical activity of the SN is under a precise regulation of the autonomous nervous system that allows it to adjust the heart rate according to the body's needs.

Studies on mammals and humans identified an anatomic or electrophysiological SN structure

constituted by the central zone or compact node (CN) and a PN zone that branch into the atrial muscle. This apparatus of 3 zones (CN-PN-atrium) guarantees the perfect function of generation and propagation of the impulse to the atrial muscle.[2]

Sinoatrial Node Central Zone

Impulse generation relies on the ability of special cells to generate a diastolic current that induces cellular depolarization. This special diastolic current is called I_f and is responsible for the pacemaker activity of the sinus node. The I_f current is generated by the spontaneous spread of sodium (Na^+) ions in the intracellular space. The molecular bases I_f are characterized by the molecular identification of the responsible family of ionic channels, the hyperpolarization-activated cyclic nucleotide-gated (HCN) channels.[3]

HCN channels are tetramers, similar to voltage-dependent potassium (K^+) channels, and this is modulated by cyclic nucleotides. There are 4 different isoforms (HCN 1–4), all expressed in different ways in the heart. In particular, isoform HCN4 is the most expressed in the SN, followed by HCN1 and HCN2, and HCN2 is the most expressed in the ventricle. HCN4 channels are greatly expressed in the cells of the sinus node and to a minor extent in the subsidiary atrial pacemakers of the AV and the bundle of His-Purkinje fibers system, whereas they are not identifiable in the normal atrial tissue that is, therefore, not able to activate spontaneously in normal conditions.[4] This is the membrane clock hypothesis of sinus node pacemaker activity, according to which a different concentration of ionic channels on the surface of the cellular membrane of the sinus node cells generates a different spontaneous depolarization current and different frequencies of intrinsic sinus automaticity. From a practical and clinical point of view in humans, it is likely that the membrane clock hypothesis can explain the ivabradine-induced bradycardia by blockage of I_f.[5] This effect is particularly useful in congestive heart failure[6] and ischemic heart disease,[7] and in any case in which the heart rate should be reduced without blocking the sympathetic drive.[8,9]

Also, the membrane clock hypothesis explains the congenital sick sinus syndrome in several families with mutations in HCN4.[10]

DiFrancesco and colleagues[11] demonstrated that catecholamines (adrenaline and noradrenaline) are able to increase the current I_f and increase the frequency of the primary pacemaker.[12] The opposite effect is determined by acetylcholine (ACh), which is responsible for the reduction of the heart rate as a result of an increase of the vagal tone.[13] These variations of the autonomic nervous system's tone balance are evident on the ECG as a respiratory sinus arrhythmia, mostly mediated by the vagal drive due to the respiratory activity (**Fig. 2**).

Paranodal Zone and Atrial Connection

Observations in animals and in humans suggest that the area around the central part of the sinus node is similar to the right atrium for some aspects and to the CN for others. The mixture of nodal and atrial cells within the PN is important because the thin layer of right atrium that lies between the PN and CN facilitates the conduction of the action potential from the SN into the right atrium. In some cases, the PN may show unstable electrical activity and consequent ectopic activity, and tachycardias are known to originate from this region.[14]

Therefore, even if the impulse's exit site is usually located in the upper part of the sinus node, the leading pacemaker site in the SN is not static and is altered in response to external factors such as sympathetic and parasympathetic stimulation; this is known as pacemaker shift in which the PN has a fundamental role. Electrocardiographically the pacemaker shift can be observed as ectopic beats or a slight modification of the initial part of the P wave.

ATRIAL ACTIVATION AND NORMAL P WAVE

Although a specific electric impulse transmission system inside the atria does not exist, there is a particular structure made of atrial muscle that allows the orderly activation of the atria. The

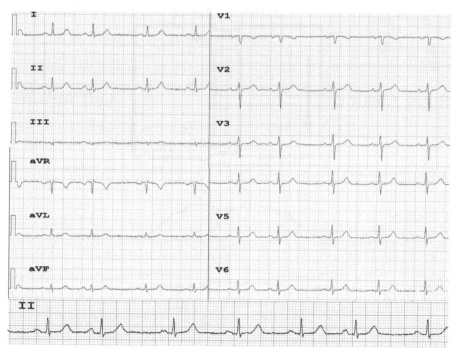

Fig. 2. Respiratory sinus arrhythmia. Phasic change in heart rate and slight modification of P wave morphology in D2 with respiration.

conduction toward the AV node is mediated by the anterior, posterior, and medial internodal tracts.

Interatrial activation occurs through a circumferential muscle band located on the anterior wall of the right atrium (BB).[15] With a conduction velocity that is almost double most of the atria, in normal hearts this bundle constitutes the major interatrial electrical connection. Transseptal conduction also occurs via other connections located around the inferior pulmonary vein (PV) and the musculature of the CS with an unclear role played by interatrial septal connections. Degeneration of BB will increase interatrial conduction time. In these circumstances, the contribution of CS and PV connections to biatrial propagation will increase with changes in P wave morphology.

The atrial activation process in the case of sinus rhythm originates from the perisinus portion of the atrial roof and extends to the anterior part and the right side of the interatrial septum until reaching the junctional region. Left atrium activation (by BB) starts 40 to 50 milliseconds after the right atrial activation and moves from the atrial roof toward the bottom. A minimal portion of left atrium made up of its posterior-inferior zones can be belatedly activated by a front coming from the CS muscle. The normal activation, therefore, can be considered as the fusion between a major activation front coming from the top through the BB and a minor terminal activation front coming from the bottom of the

interatrial septum adjacent to the CS (**Fig. 3**). This kind of activation, especially in relation to the posterior wall of the left atrium, was highlighted in a study using transesophageal electrodes,[16] as well as with electroanatomic mapping.[17]

Normal P Wave Characteristics

In the global atrial activation represented by the P wave, 3 phases can be distinguished: a first phase of right atrial activation, an intermediate phase in which both atria are activated, and a final one characterized by the activation of only the left atrium (see **Fig. 3**).

A normal atrial activation is characterized by a P wave of duration less than 120 milliseconds, an amplitude less than 0.25 mV, and an angle of the medial axis more or less equal to plus 60°. Its morphology appears rounder and positive in inferior derivations and in left precordial, where it is also possible to observe a minimal notch of the apex, an expression of the different activation timing of the 2 atria. In V1, the P wave appears positive or biphasic with positive-negative morphology (see **Fig. 2**).

IMPAIRED ATRIAL CONDUCTION OF THE SINUS NODE DEPOLARIZATION

The diffusion of the sinus node activation through the atrial conduction system can be altered both

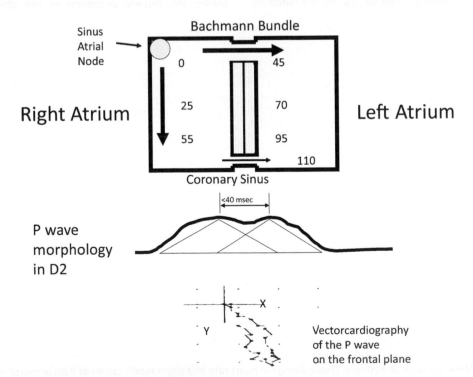

Fig. 3. Timing of the conduction system of the atria.

at the interatrial conduction (with consequent abnormalities of left atrial activation) or at the internodal conduction (with right atrial activation abnormalities).

Impaired Interatrial Conduction and Anomaly of the Left Atrial Activation

In case of normal sinus rhythm, the interatrial conduction time; that is, the interval between the right atrial activation and the beginning of the left atrial activation, is the main determinant factor for the total atrial activation. In case of severe impairment of the interatrial conduction, there is an abnormal activation of the left atrium with morphologic changes of the second part of the P wave (**Fig. 4**). The BB represents the only way the interatrial conduction is able to activate the left atrium in an orderly manner and in a top-down direction. The BB can undergo variable degrees of decreased conduction until the block.[18–20] In case of significant slowdown of the conduction on the BB, the left atrium is activated late but

with preserved top-down activation direction (see **Fig. 4**B; **Fig. 5**). The second component of the P wave will progressively get far from the first one, resulting in a pattern of P waves with longer duration (>120 ms) and forked morphology because of the presence of a second component (positive in inferior derivations) in which the apex is 40 milliseconds away from the first component. Such traces are associated to a terminal negative deflection of the P wave in V1 (0.1 mV per 40 milliseconds), and a left axial deviation of the P wave (between +45° and −30°). Those left atrial anomalies initially described in patients with mitral valve disease, also called mitral P wave, can also exist in absence of mitral valve disease and without a left atrial enlargement, merely due to a conduction delay between the 2 atria.

In advanced stages of BB conductive impairment, a complete block of the conduction can occur, a condition in which the left atrium cannot be activated from the top but only from the CS muscle (see **Fig. 4**C; **Fig. 6**). This results in a delayed backward left atrial activation

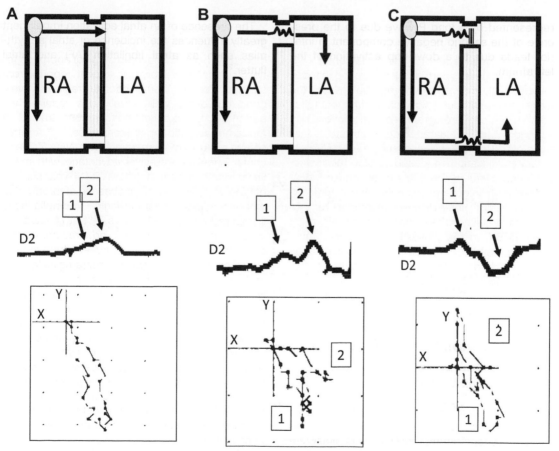

Fig. 4. Normal (*A*) and impaired (*B, C*) interatrial conduction and anomaly of the left atrial activation. (1), right atrial depolarization; (2), left atrial depolarization.

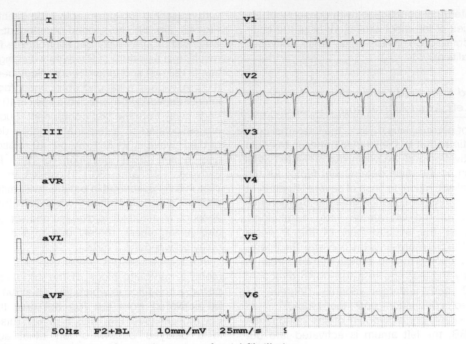

Fig. 5. Mitral P wave pattern after cardioversion of atrial fibrillation.

represented by a long P wave due to the presence of the second negative component in inferior leads due to a down-top activation of the left atrium.

The presence of an atrial activation impairment greatly influences the incidence of atrial arrhythmias such as atrial fibrillation (AF) and atrial flutter.[20]

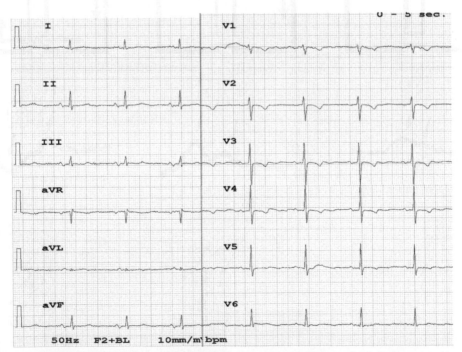

Fig. 6. P wave and complete BB block: a second negative component in inferior leads is due to a retrograde activation of the left atrium from the CS.

Right Atrial Activation Anomalies

The pressure overload of the right heart and the enlargement of the right atrium lead to an increase of the initial vectorial forces of the P wave, which have a fast and wide (>025 mV) initial component in inferior derivations and a deviation to the right on the front plane (>+75°). Besides, in V1-V2 the initial positive component of the P wave is greater than 0.15 mV (**Fig. 7**). This type of atrial activation is commonly called pulmonary P wave.

Due to the interposition of the enlarged right atrium between the right ventricle and V1, the amplitude of the QRS complex can be reduced in that derivation compared with V2, so that the amplitude of the QRS in V2 is greater than 3 times the amplitude of the QRS in V1.

ECTOPIC P WAVE

Application of multisite epicardial pace mapping with temporally implanted electrodes[21] and endocardial catheter mapping[22] has demonstrated that the 12-lead ECG can help in identifying specific sites or regions of ectopic atrial excitation within the left or right atrium.[23,24]

Fig. 8 is a simple flow chart to identify the site of origin of an ectopic atrial beat. P wave configuration in leads I and V1 are used in discriminating right atrial from left atrial foci. A negative or biphasic P wave in leads I and a positive P wave in lead V1 are helpful in predicting a left atrial site (PVs). Leads II, III, and lead aVF provide clues for differentiating superior from inferior left atrial foci. A positive P wave in II, III, or aVF indicates the superior location of the focus. Finally, a negative or biphasic P wave in lead aVL helps in predicting a left superior PV site of origin. Instead, when a right atrial origin is determined (positive P wave in lead I and negative in V1), the P wave configuration in lead aVR can differentiate activation arising from crista terminalis from those originating from tricuspid annulus or the septum. A negative P wave in lead aVR indicates the origin at crista terminalis with high sensitivity and specificity. Finally, a negative P wave in leads V5 and V6 helps in predicting a septal site of origin as opposed to a tricuspidal site of origin. Even though these simple criteria are useful, it should be underlined that analyses of surface ECG cannot supplant the need for careful endocardial mapping.

RETROGRADE ACTIVATION OF THE ATRIA

The term retrograde atrial activation, commonly known as retrograde P wave, identifies an atrial activation that sees the atria activated in the opposite mode to the spontaneous one. The identification of a true retrograde activation of the atria is extremely important in the understanding the complex electrogenetic mechanisms of an arrhythmia on the surface ECG.

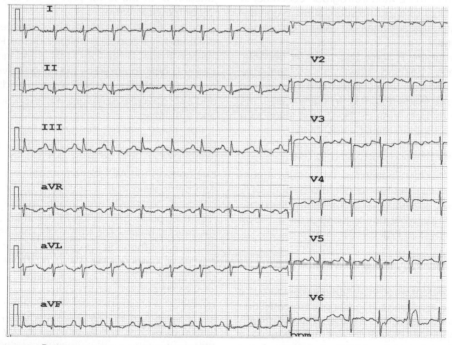

Fig. 7. Pulmonary P wave.

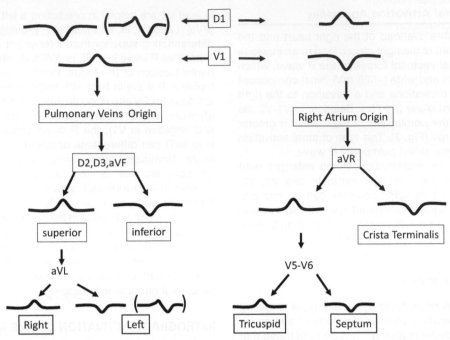

Fig. 8. Flow chart to identify the site of origin of an ectopic atrial beat.

In retrograde atrial activation, the pulse source is positioned in structures distal to the atrial mass, in the AV junction or in the ventricles, and both the atria are activated simultaneously and concentrically in down-up direction. In this context, the retrograde atrial activation must be differentiated from atrial activation that occurs in the lower part of one of the 2 atria (retrograde eccentric) in which the front of depolarization, albeit progressing retrogradely, activates an atrium before the contralateral.

The retrograde P wave has the axis perfectly vertical and pointing upwards, so that the P wave is negative in inferior leads but positive in aVR and aVL leads (**Fig. 9A**). In many cases, the simultaneous activation of the 2 atria leads to a P wave shorter than during sinus rhythm.

The correct identification of retrograde P wave can be difficult in many cases. When it falls within the QRS, this identification is technically impossible (it is not correct to identify notches of QRS as P waves), whereas inside the ventricular repolarization is possible but requires a certain level of experience (see **Fig. 9B–D**).

WANDERING PACEMAKER

In the concept of wandering pacemaker there is a progressive migration of the site of atrial activation from an anatomic site to another. This pathogenesis is supposed based on electrocardiographic observation of a progressive mutation of the

P wave from 1 form to another with at least 3 different morphologies of the P wave (**Fig. 10**).

Although many electrocardiographic aspects of wandering pacemaker are possible, the most common form to detect on the surface ECG is the migration of the rhythm between sinus node and a secondary pacemaker located in the AV junction or in the lower part of the atria (usually CS or tricuspid valve).

In the ECG, as previously described, the 2 rhythms have opposite polarity of the P wave in inferior leads. Therefore, the wandering pacemaker is characterized by the progressive positive or negative change of the P wave in leads DII, DIII, and aVF; specular variations will be present in aVR and aVL leads.

For many years, the wandering pacemaker mechanism has been attributed to the migration of the site of origin of atrial activation from the sinus node to the AV junction. Although fascinating and compelling from a graphic point of view, this concept contrasts with electrogenetic mechanisms of pulse generation in the atria. In fact, in the normal heart, cells with spontaneous automatism are not found in normal atrial tissue between the sinus node and the AV node. The electrocardiographic findings of wandering pacemaker should, therefore, be attributed to a fusion between 2 activation fronts, 1 departing from the sinus node and the other from a lower site with automatism (CS, tricuspid valve or AV junction). The gradual and progressive fusion of the 2 fronts

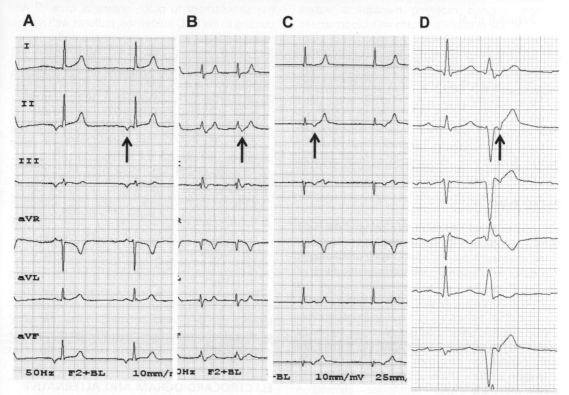

Fig. 9. Retrograde activation of the atria (*arrows*) in case of junctional rhythm (*A–C*) or ventricular ectopic beat (*D*).

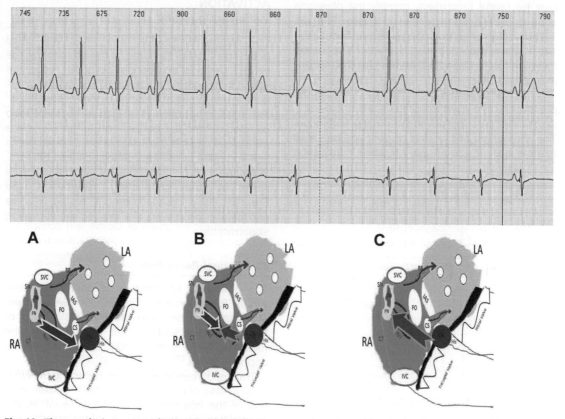

Fig. 10. The wandering pacemaker mechanism. The apparent migration of the rhythm between sinus node (*A*) and a secondary pacemaker located in the AV junction (*C*) is due to a competitive fusion between the 2 rhythms (*B*). Red arrow points to wavefront of atrial activation originating from sinus node and blue arrow points to wavefront of atrial activation originating from junctional zone.

is responsible of the progressive morphologic changes from the 2 P waves morphologies. The vagal hypertonia, which is often associated with simple breathing, plays a decisive role in the phenomenon, phasically slowing the sinus rate and thus permitting the emergence of the ectopic rhythm. The wandering pacemaker is usually a benign finding that is found in normal patients with signs of vagal hypertonia.

PACED P WAVE

The conventional site for atrial pacing is the right atrial appendage, which has also been proposed as an alternative pacing site to reduce the interatrial delay resulting from the traditional right atrial pacing. Regardless of the location of pacing, the atrial depolarization begins after a definite delay from the atrial stimulus (**Fig. 11**). The atrial depolarization that follows an atrial stimulus may be hardly visible on the surface trace, especially if there are atrial conduction disorders that make the atrial activation vectors of low amplitude and/or coincident with the next ventricular stimulation (**Fig. 12**). An esophageal recording in such cases may be useful to properly identify the presence of an atrial deflection after the atrial spike (**Fig. 13**).

The time interval from the pacing artifact to the latest signal recorded was considered to determine the total atrial activation time for the respective pacing site.

An actual objective of permanent pacing is the prevention of AF synchronizing the electrical activity of the 2 atria by advanced pacing technique. The stimulation of the atrial appendage can lead to delayed intra-atrial and interatrial conduction in many cases; alternative atrial sites have been used thinking that the beneficial effect could be a shortening of atrial activation, resulting in synchronization of left and right atrial activation. In different studies, the investigators demonstrated that BB pacing,[25] atrial septal,[26] CS os,[27] and dual site pacing (obtained by the CS and right atrial appendage)[28] shorten the duration of atrial activation compared with right atrial appendage pacing. The pacing cycle length would not have a significant impact on the respective total atrial activation time. Polarity and morphology of P wave can vary in II, III, and aVF according to the pacing site. Pacing of BB leads to a positive P wave, whereas low septal or CS os pacing leads to a negative P wave. A different spread of activation, mainly from right atrium to left atrium is produced. In this regard, it should be taken into account that P wave characteristics can be conditioned also by the intra-atrial or interatrial conduction delay eventually present in each patient.

ELECTROCARDIOGRAM AND ALTERNATIVE METHODS FOR THE STUDY OF ATRIAL ACTIVATION
Vectorcardiography

The vectorcardiographic analysis of the atrial activation highlights some aspects such as the various vectorial components of the P wave, the global morphology, the interval, and spatial distribution of the atrial activation. In normal conditions, the atrial conduction is a unique vectorial loop directed toward the bottom and to the left on the front plane and it is the fusion of the 2 components (left and right) of the atrial activation (see **Fig. 4**A). When the morphology of the P wave changes as a result of atrial conduction disturbance (see **Fig. 4**B, C), vectorcardiography of the P wave can clearly represent the respective activation abnormalities.

Esophageal Recording

The possibility of using endoesophageal electrodes for recording atrial ECG is well-known. The contiguity between the terminal portion of the esophagus and the left atrium allows the recording of wide and clear left atrial depolarizations.[29]

Transesophageal recordings detecting the electrical activity of the left atrium allow the determination of the interatrial conduction, meant as the interval between the beginning of the atrial activation measured on the surface ECG and the local atrial depolarization measured at the endoesophageal level (**Fig. 14**).

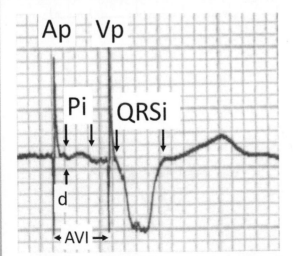

Fig. 11. Paced P wave. Ap, atrial pacing; d, delay of activation from Ap to Pi; AVI, atrioventricular interval; Pi, induced P wave; QRSi, induced QRS; Vp, ventricular pacing.

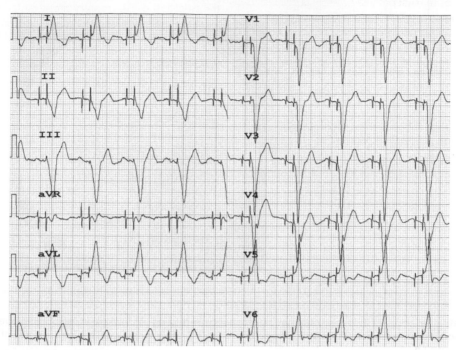

Fig. 12. AV pacing. Conventional ECG.

The use of multiple consecutive bipolar derivations via multipolar catheters allows the mapping of the activation direction of the left atrium. In a study of 30 subjects in sinus rhythm after electrical cardioversion of persistent atrial fibrillation,[16] atrial activation was studied by combining 12-lead ECG and multipolar esophageal recordings. Proximal and distal esophageal recording characterize the longitudinal direction of activation of the posterior left atrium (**Fig. 15**).

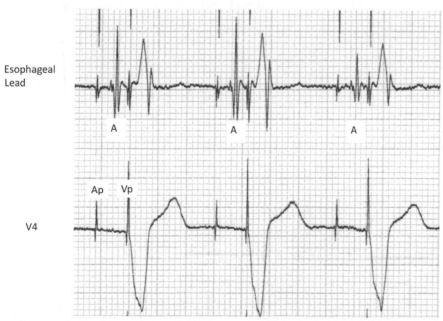

Fig. 13. AV pacing. On the lead V4 the atrial induced depolarization is not clear, whereas on the esophageal recording the atrial depolarization (A) is well-evident.

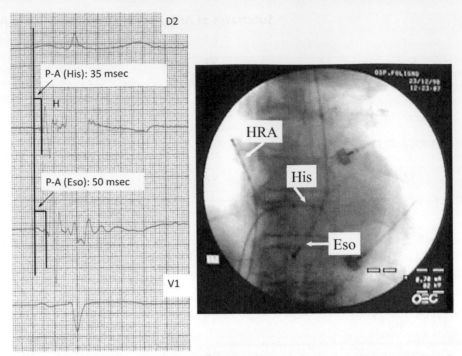

Fig. 14. Left atrial origin of the signal obtained by esophageal recording. PA interval at esophageal level is significantly longer then the classical PA interval recorded at Hisian level. Eso, esophageal lead; His, bundle of His; HRA, hight right atrium.

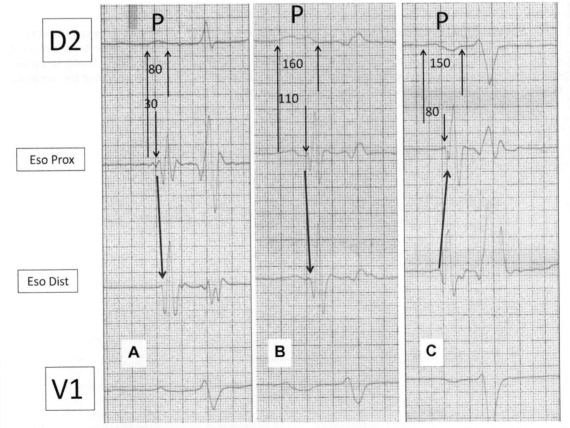

Fig. 15. Left atrial posterior wall recording by a multipolar oesophageal lead (Eso Prox and Eso Dist) in case of normal atrial activation (*A*), BB delay (*B*) and BB block (*C*). P wave duration is 80, 160, 150 msec respectively in (*A*), (*B*), (*C*). Interatrial conduction time is 30, 110, 80 msec respectively in (*A*), (*B*), (*C*). The dark arrows indicate the direction of activation of the left atrial posterior wall.

THE SUBSTRATES OF ATRIAL ARRHYTHMIAS: CORRELATION BETWEEN SPECIAL STRUCTURAL BASES AND THE POTENTIAL DEVELOPMENT OF ARRHYTHMIAS
Ionic Channels, Anatomic Structures, and Innervation

Atrial anatomy is very complex, it includes multiple orifices; trabeculated myocardium; overlapping fibromuscular layers; and, in some locations, a mixture of different tissues. As an example, in the PVs, sleeves of myocardial tissue provide a sphincter like function and are deeply embedded within the vein anatomic structure. A further complexity is added by the migration of automatic cells during embryogenesis from primitive embryogenic tubes to specific anatomic sites in the fully developed heart. This intricate development of tissues with different electrophysiological properties can offer multiple substrates to the 3 mechanisms underlying all arrhythmias. Abnormal automaticity, triggered activity, and re-entry have all been documented in humans, with more than one mechanism often coexisting, rendering clinical understanding of the arrhythmia very challenging.

Evidence of abnormal impulse formation, either as triggered activity or as abnormal automaticity, is difficult to document in the normal atria due to the sporadic nature of this mechanism. On the contrary, discontinuous propagation, also referred as anisotropy, which underlies the mechanism of re-entry, is evident even during sinus rhythm. Fractionated electrogram, double potentials, fibrosis, and continuous electrical activity, all considered to be hallmarks of anisotropy, are easily recorded in normal atria[30] and more frequently detected in patients with documented flutter or fibrillation[31,32] (Fig. 16).

Both atria are extensively innervated and it is well-known that sympathetic and parasympathetic discharges markedly affect the electrophysiological properties of every myocardial cell.[33] The interplay between the 2 arms of the autonomic nervous system and their role in arrhythmia's genesis is still an area of fertile speculation.

Acquired pathologic conditions, such as scars or dilatation, and the physiologic process of aging, can alter atrial functional properties. Decreased cell to cell contact, accumulation of fibrous tissue, and alteration of channel expression and function all favor an arrhythmogenic milieu already present in normal atria.

Cardiac Nervous System

From its origin at the stellate ganglia, the cervical sympathetic trunks, and the recurrent laryngeal nerves or the vagi, the cardiac nervous system

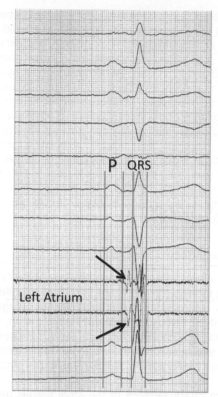

Fig. 16. Fractionated atrial electrical activity after atrial fibrillation. Left atrial recording at esophageal level after cardioversion of AF shows delayed atrial potential well beyond the end of the surface P wave (*arrows*).

ends with diffuse arborization at the cardiac levels. These are evident in many macroscopic and microscopic ganglionated plexi embedded in pericardial fat and distributed in both atria in a discrete and nonuniform manner.[34] The interplay of sympathetic and parasympathetic efferents is very complex, and it is not surprising that the role of the autonomic nervous system in the induction and maintenance of atrial arrhythmias is still not fully understood. Both in animals and humans, the effects of vagal stimulation are more relevant than those of sympathetic stimulation in promoting atrial tachyarrhythmias.[35] ACh, released during vagal stimulation, produces shortening of action potential and of refractory period, increasing the heterogeneity normally present across the atrial wall and creating a substrate for re-entry.[36] In dogs, AF could be induced by either vagal stimulation or systemic infusion of ACh without electrical stimulation of the atria. In humans, stimulation of the ganglionated plexi around the PVs, an area considered to be determinant in the initiation and maintenance of AF, can trigger ectopy and AF.[37]

Furthermore a strong relationship exists between vagal stimuli and specific pathologic conditions, such as nocturnal AF, AF in athletes, and patients with gastrointestinal disorders. Clinical studies aimed at defining the role of the autonomic system in human AF have attempted to eliminate, mostly with radiofrequency ablation, the ganglia localized in proximity of the PVs to assess whether a reduction of vagal stimulation can prevent AF. The results suggest that vagal stimulation mostly facilitates induction and maintenance of these arrhythmias. AF, in fact, cannot be prevented by stand-alone plexi ablation because elimination of ganglia during standard ablation for AF prolongs freedom from atrial arrhythmias.[38]

Automaticity

Premature atrial complexes (PACs) and sustained atrial tachycardia are often the clinical manifestations of abnormal automaticity or triggered activity.[39] Although PACs are very common, sustained atrial tachycardia is rarely documented in clinical practice; however, both constitute a fundamental pathogenetic mechanism in the initiation of AF.[40]

The characteristics of the atrial tissues generating PACs and atrial tachycardias are not uniform nor well-documented, whereas their anatomic location has been better characterized (**Fig. 17**). Seeding of automatic cells during embryogenesis has been postulated in human and animal studies. A specific antigen, HNK-1, expressed by tissue with automatic properties has been identified within human embryonic structures that will develop into the PVs, coronary sinus, and crista terminalis.[41] In an animal model, cells with nodal characteristics have been documented around both tricuspid and mitral annuli. It is unclear whether these findings represent spurious seeding during the complex process of cardiac development or the physiologic establishment of subsidiary pacemaker centers to maintain cardiac excitation in case of sinus node failure. However, the concept of a widely distributed pacemaker system with a dominant sinus node and a large number of subsidiary pacemakers has been validated in many studies.[42] Additionally, the sites of abnormal ectopic atrial tachycardia and the locations of these extranodal atrial pacemakers are frequently identical. It is conceivable, therefore, that under the influence of some cardiac pathologic condition, these extranodal pacemaker cells can escape cholinergic control, acquire increased adrenergic sensitivity, or can develop an entrance but not an exit block. .Further evidence supporting automaticity in these sites comes from studies showing, in humans and dogs, extension of muscle fibers into the fibrous leaflet of the anterior mitral valve. These cells can exhibit spontaneous activity or repetitive discharges when exposed to catecholamines or stretch. The electrophysiological characteristics of the myocytes in this area exhibit

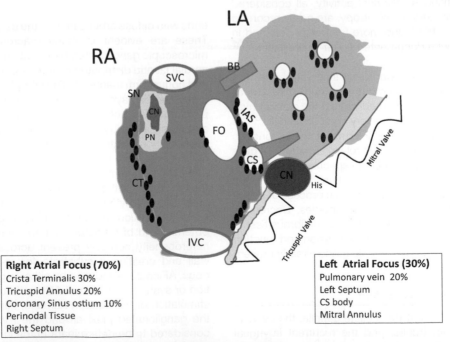

Right Atrial Focus (70%)	Left Atrial Focus (30%)
Crista Terminalis 30%	Pulmonary vein 20%
Tricuspid Annulus 20%	Left Septum
Coronary Sinus ostium 10%	CS body
Perinodal Tissue	Mitral Annulus
Right Septum	

Fig. 17. Right and left atrial ectopic beats and tachycardias location.

slow-rising action potential and pacemaker activity similar to sinus node or AV node cells.

The crista terminalis remains the site of origin of up to two-thirds of right ATs, as well as the physiologic location of the sinus node. This region is characterized by a marked anisotropy due to poor transverse cell-to-cell coupling, which explains the fundamental role the crista terminalis plays in the genesis of atrial flutter. Furthermore, nodal cells extend for variable length along the long axis of this structure. The combination of automatic tissue with relative cellular uncoupling may favor the emergence of abnormal automaticity by decreasing normal electronic inhibition of phase 4 depolarization exerted by myocytes in close contact.

Additionally, myocardial cells that normally do not exhibit automatic features can, under specific circumstances, acquire membrane instability, leading to spontaneous electrical discharges. In every location where this occurs, a mixture of fibroblast and myocytes is present because different histologic cardiac structures often merge into each other. Automatic foci have been described clinically in the superior vena cava and in the myocardial fibers connecting this structure to the right atrium. Convincing evidence of phase 4 depolarization, accompanied by the initiation of automatic activity within these fibers, offers a good mechanistic explanation for the arrhythmias.

Spontaneous firing from PVs was the initial observation leading to current understanding and therapy for AF.[40] Despite this clinical observation and extensive reconfirmation of this finding, a direct demonstration of spontaneous automaticity in normal human PV cardiomyocytes is lacking. On the contrary, in human embryos and in animal experiments with drug infusion, atrial distension, or rapid atrial firing, triggered and abnormal PVs automatic activity has been consistently demonstrated. Histologic studies have shown that, in normal hearts, atrial myocardium extends deeply in the PVs in the form of disconnected strands surrounded by many fibroblasts.[43] The close contact of atrial cardiomyocytes and fibroblasts leads to anisotropies, due to heterocellular electrical coupling and to a reduction in myocyte's resting membrane potential. This is followed by spontaneous triggered activity with automatic discharges. This mechanism could explain the arrhythmic discharges, previously mentioned, observed in myocytes embedded in fibrous tissue in both the superior vena cava and mitral valve.[44]

In summary, both excessive automatic or triggered activity seem to underlie the mechanism of atrial tachycardias. Physiologic subsidiary pacemakers located in specific anatomic sites can, under pathologic conditions, increase their resting rate. The inevitable contact between fibroblasts and myocytes changes their electrophysiological characteristics, predisposing the latter to automatism and leading to the emergence of arrhythmic foci.

Re-entry

The theory of anatomic re-entry[45] predicts the presence of areas of different refractoriness and of an anatomic pathway capable of accommodating the entire re-entrant circuit. The length of the pathway is fixed because it is determined by anatomy, so the viability of re-entry is determined by the product of conduction velocity and tissue refractoriness. For anatomic re-entrant circuits to exist, an excitable interval or gap must exist between the end of refractoriness of a cycle and the beginning of excitation of the next. The right atrium anatomy is perfectly predisposed to initiate and maintain typical atrial flutter, the most common clinical re-entry. Anisotropy due to different fiber orientation[46] is common and is particularly evident at the crista terminalis and at the eustachian ridge between the isthmus and the CS os. The crista terminalis increases its physiologic anisotropy, possibly during sinus rhythm but more so when exposed to premature beats or high stimulation rates. This leads to the complete transverse uncoupling of conduction and creates a functional block to impulse propagation.[47] Therefore, the crista terminalis with the eustachian ridge as a continuation, and the orifices of inferior vena cava and superior vena cava, represent the posterior boundary of atrial flutter and creates 2 distinct wavefronts of activation. One wavefront propagates along the inferoposterior wall of the right atrium while, more anteriorly, a second wavefront is forced around the tricuspid valve. The crista terminalis, by isolating these 2 wavefronts, maintains the viability of the circuit, preventing a premature depolarization, or short circuiting, of the anterior wall by the inferoposterior wavefront. The tricuspid annulus constitutes the anterior boundary of the circuit, delimiting the virtual ring of myocardium supporting the typical atrial flutter circuit (**Fig. 18**).

An area of nonuniform myocardial trabeculation is present, in normal hearts, at the lower level of the triangle of Koch and the CS os, potentially constituting the area of slow conduction necessary in the induction of re-entry. Rate-dependent conduction delay and unidirectional block in the low right atrium between the inferior vena cava, tricuspid annulus, and CS os was demonstrated during rapid pacing, with induction of clockwise and counter-clockwise typical flutter.

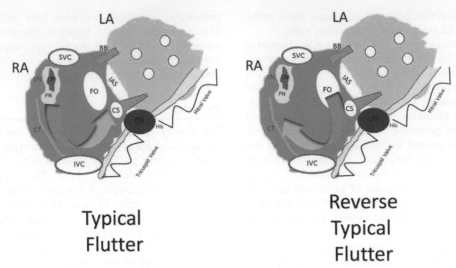

Fig. 18. Typical atrial flutter with clockwise and counter-clockwise rotation around the tricuspid valve.

AF, the most common atrial arrhythmia, remains also the least well-characterized. Several studies suggest that AF is likely to be a common manifestation of several arrhythmic mechanisms. The variable interplay between rapid firing triggers and different anatomic substrates[41] seems to be a reasonable model explaining most of the features of AF. In the early stages of AF, the combination of fast discharging atrial focus with anisotropic tissues unable to support 1:1 propagation could explain the emergence of fibrillatory conduction, characterized with wave-breaks and appearance of spiral waves.[48] In the more chronic forms of AF, histologic changes and derangement of electrophysiological properties create the substrate for persistent arrhythmia.[49] In normal hearts, and more so in aging, dilated, or scarred atria, the emergence of extensive, localized anisotropy predisposes these chambers to fibrillatory conduction and multiple re-entry wavelets. The role of PVs myocardial sleeves in the genesis of AF has been the focus of many reports. Animal and human studies have shown the dual role of PVs as initiators of automatic discharges and substrates for microreentry.[50] Isolated PV myocytes, demonstrating pacemaker activity and triggered after depolarizations with development of ionic currents, mimicking sinus node cells were observed in animal studies.[51] It is likely that altered electronic inhibition in strands of muscle fibers embedded in different histologic tissue increases the resting membrane potential, contributing to the propensity for automaticity of these structures. Furthermore, there is abundant evidence that the proximal PVs contain areas of abrupt changes in the fibers' orientation. This creates anisotropic conduction and prolonged refractoriness, generating a substrate

for re-entry in response to premature stimulation. This re-entry is a functional re-entry occurring, differently from typical flutter, in the absence of anatomic obstacles.[52] The marked tissue anisotropy shown by the PVs is not peculiar to these structures. Both atria also contain multiple interwoven muscular bundles with abrupt changes in fiber orientation, creating areas of marked anisotropy (see previous discussion). These areas, when stimulated at high frequencies, become functional obstacles to conduction, generating unidirectional blocks and functional re-entries, leading to fibrillatory conduction. Areas that have been shown in animal models and human studies to be relevant to the origination and maintenance of AF include the posterior left atrial wall, the CS, the pectinate muscles, and the ligament of Marshall. These studies also strongly suggest that at a specific stimulation frequency, the normally organized 1:1 conduction gives way to the formation of rotors and wave brakes degenerating into clinical AF. This mechanism explains very well how a stable rhythm, such as atrial tachycardia or atrial flutter, on reaching a critical cycle length leads to AF.

In summary, the anatomic features of the atria that evolved to ensure optimal emptying and effective activation of wavefront propagation became the unwitting cause of stable or unstable arrhythmias.

REFERENCES

1. Spach MS, Dolber PC, Heidlage FJ. Interaction of inhomogeneities of repolarization with anisotropic propagation in dog atria. Circ Res 1989;65:1612–31.
2. Chandler NJ, Greener ID, Tellez JO, et al. Molecular architecture of the human sinus node insights into

the function of the cardiac pacemaker. Circulation 2009;119:1562–75.

3. Ludwig A, Zong X, Jeglitsch M, et al. A family of hyperpolarization-activated mammalian cation channels. Nature 1998;393:587–91.

4. Nof E, Antzelevitch C, Glikson M. The contribution of HCN4 to normal sinus node function in humans and animal models. Pacing Clin Electrophysiol 2010;33: 100–6.

5. Bucchi A, Baruscotti M, DiFrancesco D. Current-dependent block of rabbit sino-atrial node if channels by ivabradine. J Gen Physiol 2002;120:1–13.

6. Swedberg K, Komajda M, Böhm M, et al, SHIFT Investigators. Ivabradine and outcomes in chronic heart failure (SHIFT): a randomised placebo-controlled study. Lancet 2010;376:875–85.

7. Fasullo S, Cannizzaro S, Maringhini G, et al. Comparison of ivabradine versus metoprolol in early phases of reperfused anterior myocardial infarction with impaired left ventricular function: preliminary findings. J Card Fail 2009;15:856–63.

8. DiFrancesco D, Camm JA. Heart rate lowering by specific and selective if current inhibition with ivabradine: a new therapeutic perspective in cardiovascular disease. Drugs 2004;64:1757–65.

9. Heusch G. Pleiotropic action(s) of the bradycardic agent ivabradine: cardiovascular protection beyond heart rate reduction. Br J Pharmacol 2008;155: 970–1.

10. Dobrzynski H, Boyett MR, Anderson RH. New insights into pacemaker activity: promoting understanding of sick sinus syndrome. Circulation 2007; 115:1921–32.

11. DiFrancesco D, Ferroni A, Mazzanti M, et al. Properties of the hyperpolarizing-activated current sino-atrial node. J Physiol 1986;377:61–88.

12. DiFrancesco D, Tromba C. Inhibition of the hyperpolarization-activated current (if) induced by acetylcholine in rabbit sino-atrial node myocytes. J Physiol 1988;405:477–91.

13. DiFrancesco D, Ducouret P, Robinson RB. Muscarinic modulation of cardiac rate at low acetylcholine concentrations. Science 1989;243:669–71.

14. Medi C, Kalman JM, Ling LH, et al. Atrial electrical and structural remodeling associated with longstanding pulmonary hypertension and right ventricular hypertrophy in humans. J Cardiovasc Electrophysiol 2012;23:614–20.

15. De Ponti R, Ho S, Salerno-Uriarte JA, et al. Electroanatomic analysis of sinus impulse propagation in normal human atria. J Cardiovasc Electrophysiol 2002;13(1):1–10.

16. Bagliani G, Michelucci A, Angeli F. Atrial activation analysis by surface P wave and multipolar esophageal recording after cardioversion of persistent atrial fibrillation. Pacing Clin Electrophysiol 2003; 26:1178–88.

17. Markides V, Schilling RJ, Ho SY, et al. Characterization of left atrial activation in the intact human heart. Circulation 2003;107:733–9.

18. Bayés de Luna A, Guindo J, Vinolas X, et al. Third degree (advanced) interatrial block. G Ital Cardiol 1998;28(Suppl 1):26–9.

19. Jairath UC, Spodick DH. Exceptional prevalence of interatrial block in a general hospital population. Clin Cardiol 2001;24(8):548–50.

20. Michelucci A, Padeletti L, Chelucci A, et al. Influence of age, lead axis, frequency of arrhythmic episodes, and atrial dimensions on P wave-triggered signal-averaged ECG in patients with lone paroxysmal atrial fibrillation. Pacing Clin Electrophysiol 1996;19:758–67.

21. MacLean WHA, Karp RB, Kouchoukos NT, et al. P waves during ectopic atrial rhythms in man. A study utilizing atrial pacing with fixed electrodes. Circulation 1975;52:426–34.

22. SippensGroenewegen A, Peeters HA, Jessurun ER, et al. Body surface mapping during pacing at multiple sites in the human atrium. P wave morphology of ectopic right atrial activation. Circulation 1998;97: 369–80.

23. Tada H, Nogami A, Naito S, et al. Simple electrocardiographic criteria for identifying the site of origin of focal right atrial tachycardia. Pacing Clin Electrophysiol 1998;21(11 Pt 2):2431–9.

24. Morton JB, Sanders P, Das A, et al. Focal atrial tachycardia arising from the tricuspid annulus: electrophysiologic and electrocardiographic characteristics. J Cardiovasc Electrophysiol 2001;12:653–9.

25. Bailin SJ, Adler S, Giudici M. Prevention of chronic atrial fibrillation by pacing in the region of Bachmann's bundle: results of a multicenter randomized trial. J Cardiovasc Electrophysiol 2001;12:912–7.

26. Padeletti L, Porciani MC, Michelucci A, et al. Interatrial septum pacing: a new approach to prevent recurrent atrial fibrillation. J Interv Card Electrophysiol 1999;3:35–43.

27. Delfaut P, Saksena S, Prakash A, et al. Long-term outcome of patients with drug-refractory atrial flutter and fibrillation after single- and dual-site right atrial pacing for arrhythmia prevention. J Am Coll Cardiol 1998;32:1900–8.

28. D'Allonnes GR, Pavin D, Leclercq C, et al. Long-term effects of biatrial synchronous pacing to prevent drug-refractory atrial tachyarrhythmia: a nine year experience. J Cardiovasc Electrophysiol 2000; 11(10):1081–91.

29. Bagliani G, Meniconi L, Raggi F, et al. Left origin of the atrial esophageal signal as recorded in the pacing site. Pacing Clin Electrophysiol 1998;21(1 Pt 1): 18–24.

30. Cassidy DM, Vassallo JA, Miller JM, et al. Endocardial catheter mapping in patients in sinus rhythm: relationship to underlying heart disease and ventricular arrhythmias. Circulation 1986;73:645–52.

31. Centurion OA, Fukatani M, Konoe A, et al. Electro-physiological abnormalities of the atrial muscle in patients with sinus node dysfunction without tachy-arrhythmias. Int J Cardiol 1992;37(1):41–50.

32. Tanigawa M, Fukatani M, Konoe A, et al. Prolonged and fractionated right atrial electrograms during si-nus rhythm in patients with paroxysmal atrial fibrilla-tion and sick sinus node syndrome. J Am Coll Cardiol 1991;17(2):403–8.

33. Janes RD, Brandys JC, Hopkins DA, et al. Anatomy of human extrinsic cardiac nerves and ganglia. Am J Cardiol 1986;57:299–309.

34. Liu L, Nattel S. Differing sympathetic and vagal effects on atrial fibrillation in dogs: role of refractori-ness heterogeneity. Am J Physiol 1997;273:H805–16.

35. Zipes DP, Mihalick MJ, Robbins GT. Effects of selec-tive vagal and stellate ganglion stimulation on atrial refractoriness. Cardiovasc Res 1974;8:647–55.

36. Coumel P. Autonomic influences in atrial tachyarrhyth-mias. J Cardiovasc Electrophysiol 1996;7:999–1007.

37. Danik S, Neuzil P, d'Avila A, et al. Evaluation of cath-eter ablation of periatrial ganglionic plexi in patients with atrial fibrillation. Am J Cardiol 2008;102:578–83.

38. Chen SA, Chiang CE, Yang CJ, et al. Sustained atrial tachycardia in adult patients. Electrophysiological characteristics, pharmacological response, possible mechanisms, and effects of radiofrequency ablation. Circulation 1994;90:1262–78.

39. Scheinman MM, Basu D, Hollenberg M. Electro-physiologic studies in patients with persistent atrial tachycardia. Circulation 1994;50:266–73.

40. Haïssaguerre M, Jaïs P, Shah DC, et al. Sponta-neous initiation of atrial fibrillation by ectopic beats originating in the pulmonary veins. N Engl J Med 1998;339(10):659–66.

41. Blom NA, Gittenberger-de Groot AC, DeRuiter MC, et al. Development of the cardiac conduction tissue in human embryos using HNK-1 antigen expression possible relevance for understanding of abnormal atrial automaticity. Circulation 1999;99:800–6.

42. Boineau JP, Canavan TE, Schuessler RB, et al. Demonstration of a widely distributed atrial pace-maker complex in the human heart. Circulation 1988;77(6):1221–37.

43. Saito T, Waki K, Becker AE. Left atrial myocardial extension onto pulmonary veins in humans: anatomic observations relevant for atrial arrhyth-mias. J Cardiovasc Electrophysiol 2000;11:888–94.

44. Rohr S. Myofibroblasts in diseased hearts: new players in cardiac arrhythmias? Heart Rhythm 2009;6(6):848–56.

45. Moe GK. Evidence for reentry as a mechanism of cardiac arrhythmias. Rev Physiol Biochem Pharma-col 1975;72:55–81.

46. Spach MS, Miller WT Jr, Dolber PC, et al. The func-tional role of structural complexities in the propaga-tion of depolarization in the atrium of the dog: cardiac conduction disturbances due to discontinu-ities of effective axial resistivity. Circ Res 1982;50:175–91.

47. Schumacher B, Jung W, Schmidt H, et al. Transverse conduction capabilities of the crista terminalis in pa-tients with atrial flutter and atrial fibrillation. J Am Coll Cardiol 1999;34(2):363–73.

48. Nattel S, Shiroshita-Takeshita A, Bianca JJM, et al. Mechanisms of atrial fibrillation: lessons from animal models. Prog Cardiovasc Dis 2005;48:9–28.

49. Allessie M, Ausma J, Schotten U. Electrical, contrac-tile, structural remodeling during atrial fibrillation. Cardiovasc Res 2002;54:230–46.

50. Hocini M, Ho SY, Kawara T, et al. Electrical conduc-tion in canine pulmonary veins electrophysiological and anatomic correlation. Circulation 2002;105:2442–8.

51. Hamabe A, Okuyama Y, Miyauchi Y, et al. Correla-tion between anatomy and electrical activation in canine pulmonary veins. Circulation 2003;107:1550–5.

52. Vaquero M, Calvo D, Jalife J. Cardiac fibrillation: from ion channels to rotors in the human heart. Heart Rhythm 2008;5:872–9.

Arrhythmias Originating in the Atria

Fabio Leonelli, MD[a], Giuseppe Bagliani, MD[b,c],*, Giuseppe Boriani, MD[d], Luigi Padeletti, MD[e,f]

KEYWORDS

- Atrial arrhythmias • Atrial flutter • Atrial fibrillation • Atrial tachycardia • Scar-related arrhythmias
- ECG

KEY POINTS

- ECG, thanks to its low cost and accessibility, remains a valuable tool in the diagnosis of arrhythmias.
- The relationship between ECG morphology and atrial activation, as well as wavefront progression, has been clarified by intracardiac mapping.
- The ECG definition of atrial arrhythmias is based on recognition of specific patterns related to definite sequences of atrial activation.
- Atrial flutter (AFL), with its main variants, is a complex macro-reentry. Its mechanism and activation path can often be identified by an attentive analysis of the ECG tracing.
- The site of origin of focal atrial tachycardias due to enhanced automaticity or micro-reentry can be reliably identified on ECG although their mechanism remains often unknown.
- Despite that atrial fibrillation's origin, persistence, and mechanisms have been largely explained, these advances have not translated into a more meaningful analysis of the ECG of this arrhythmia.

INTRODUCTION

ECG and Electrophysiology: The Advantage of Intracardiac Recordings

ECG remains the most useful noninvasive tool in the diagnosis of atrial tachyarrhythmias (**Figs. 1–3**). The diagnostic criteria of each arrhythmia have been elucidated over many years of observation and deductive analysis; with the advent of animal studies, arrhythmias' mechanisms were also fully defined. The concepts of reentry, abnormal automaticity, and triggered activity were postulated and demonstrated in animal studies over the past 50 years. These observations were extrapolated to human arrhythmias when clinical and experimental data coincided. Human intracardiac recordings, followed by sophisticated 3-D reconstructions of cardiac electrical activity, have opened the doors to confirmations and revisions of previous understanding of arrhythmias. Abnormal automaticity and triggered activity are difficult to diagnose even during electrophysiology studies and require assessing the response to multiple intravenous drugs and, at times, monophasic action potential recordings. There are some observations made during invasive studies also present during ECG analysis that may help differentiate between these 2 mechanisms. The clinical usefulness of this information is debatable

No relevant conflicts to disclose.

[a] Cardiology Department James A. Haley Veterans' Hospital, University South Florida, 13000 Bruce B Down Boulevard, Tampa 33612, FL, USA; [b] Arrhythmology Unit, Cardiology Department, Foligno General Hospital, Via Massimo Arcamone, 06034 Foligno (PG), Italy; [c] Cardiovascular Diseases Department, University of Perugia, Piazza Menghini 1, 06129 Perugia Italy; [d] Cardiology Department, Modena University Hospital, University of Modena and Reggio Emilia, Via Università, 4, 41121 Modena, Italy; [e] Heart and Vessels Department, University of Florence, Largo Brambilla, 3, 50134 Florence, Italy; [f] IRCCS Multimedica, Cardiology Department, Via Milanese, 300, 20099 Sesto San Giovanni, Italy

* Corresponding author. Via Centrale Umbra 17, Spello, Perugia 06038, Italy.
E-mail address: giuseppe.bagliani@tim.it

Card Electrophysiol Clin 9 (2017) 383–409
http://dx.doi.org/10.1016/j.ccep.2017.05.002
1877-9182/17/© 2017 Elsevier Inc. All rights reserved.

cardiacEP.theclinics.com

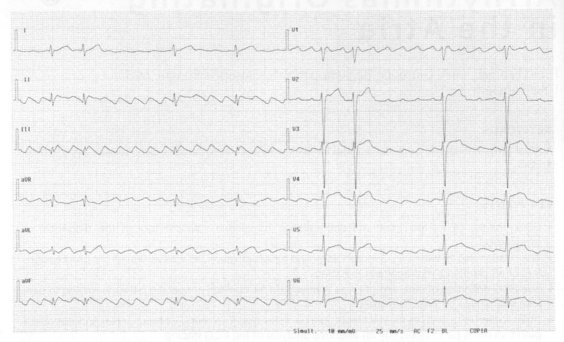

Fig. 1. AFL, common type, with the typical sawtooth pattern in the inferior leads.

because there are no consistent data supporting a specific drug regimen based on the mechanism of either arrhythmia. The study and characterization of reentry, on the other hand, has been one of the most rewarding electrophysiologic endeavors. From its initial concept in a ring of jellyfish to the

analysis of fibrillatory conduction in animals and humans, reentry has been defined and understood in almost its entirety. Transfer of this knowledge to the realm of ECG, has helped understand, for example, the genesis of ECG waveforms during typical flutter and better define reentrant atrial

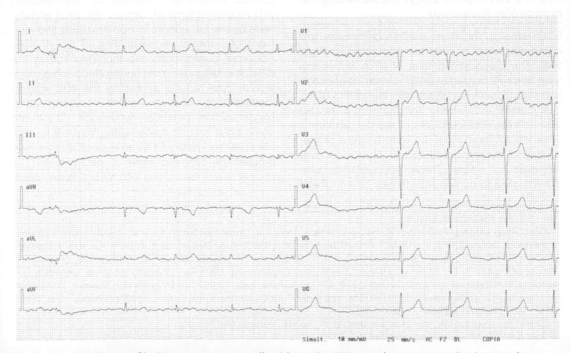

Fig. 2. Atrial fibrillation: fibrillation waves are well evident, the QRS complexes are completely irregular.

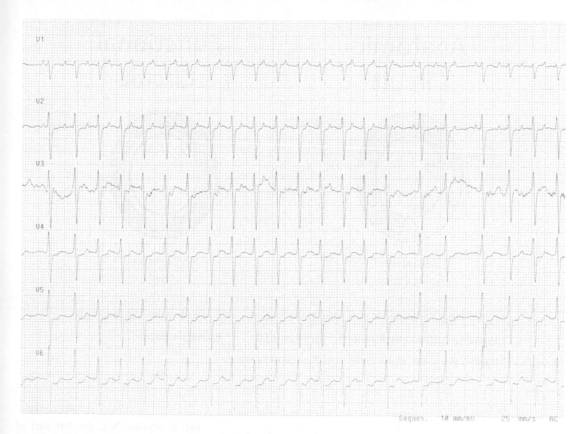

Fig. 3. Atrial tachycardia: a tachycardic fast atrial activity is clearly evident; the P waves are separated by an iso-electric line. See **Fig. 16** for more details.

tachycardias. As always is the case, deeper knowledge has generated further questions and highlighted the diagnostic limitations of the standard ECG.

From Intracardiac Recording to Surface ECG: A Confirmation of Arrhythmia's Mechanisms

AFL is, because of its stability, ease of induction, and frequent occurrence in clinical practice, the arrhythmia that has generated the majority of knowledge of reentry. Sir Thomas Lewis, integrating clinical observations with ECG tracings and animal studies, led the way, at the beginning of the last century, to the definition of the reentrant pathway. Cardiac electrophysiology confirmed and expanded this basic knowledge to humans, defining 2 types of reentry (**Fig. 4**): anatomic or fixed and functional. In the former, the role of obstacles to conduction, either anatomic or scars; the importance of a slow conducting region; and the criteria necessary for the diagnosis of reentry were provided by a series of seminal studies approximately 50 years later.

With the advent of 3-D mapping during electrophysiology study, the visualization of the entire reentrant pathway was obtained, guiding target destruction with radiofrequency energy of essential portions of the circuit and permanent interruption of the reentry. Additionally, the detailed intracardiac description of the activation wavefront has allowed correlating this information to the ECG components of the flutter (F) waves during its atrial progression. These observations have, therefore, led to the ECG diagnostic criteria of most flutters. Constant reentry engaging both atria is manifested as a continuous activity without a discernable baseline in the 12-lead ECG (see **Fig. 1**). The same ECG observations allow predicting not only isthmus dependency, distinguishing typical flutters versus atypical flutter (**Fig. 5**), but also ascertaining the direction of its rotation around anatomic obstacles, clockwise (CW) (**Fig. 6**) or counterclockwise (CCW) (**Fig. 7**).

When compared with anatomic reentry, functional reentry is less well understood although most of its mechanism is well defined. Both types of reentry share the same principles. Either type

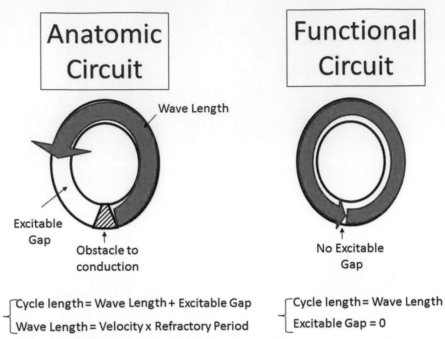

Fig. 4. Anatomic and functional characteristics of the reentry circuits.

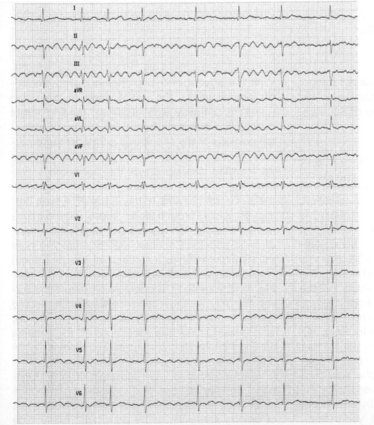

Fig. 5. Atypical AFL, the left part of the figure, degenerates into atrial fibrillation.

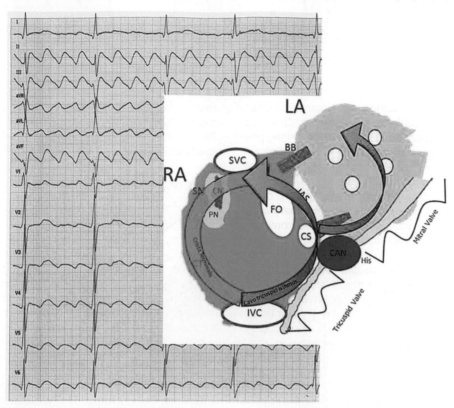

Fig. 6. CCW AFL: anatomic and ECG correlations. CAN, compact atrioventricular node; CN, central node; FO, fossa ovalis; HIS, his bundle; IAS, interatrial septum; PN, perinodal zone; SN, sinus node.

requires tissue with different electrophysiologic properties favoring slow conduction and block of propagation, and each type also necessitates excitable myocardium ahead of its leading wavefront. In the anatomic or fixed form, anatomy or scars provide the milieu and determines the reentrant pathway. In functional reentry, when an activation wavefront encounters an area of tissue in different stages of repolarization, it loses its stable progression and break into regions of block or nonuniform, slower conduction velocity. In the presence of increased tissue heterogeneity, the wave breaks generates either multiple wavelets or an initial rotational propagation assuming the configuration of a rotor. Either way, eventually multiple wavelets are produced, quickly degenerating into fibrillatory conduction (see **Fig. 5**). Endocardial recordings register a continuing disorganized activity defying interpretation. Similarly, the ECG reflects continuous activation of mostly low voltage without a recognizable P wave. Although periods of increased electrical organization, possibly reflecting the temporary formation of a rotor, may be seen as a larger, more defined P wave, the overall impression is one of profound disorganization.

Accurate intracardiac mapping of regular atrial arrhythmias has greatly helped understanding of their mechanism of origin and propagation. Combining this information with analysis of the ECG has allowed expanding the diagnostic capabilities of this tool. In cases of atrial tachycardia, for example, intracardiac recording has helped better define this arrhythmia and identify the overlapping features with macro-reentrant flutter. Electrophysiologic studies have also identified the mechanisms of atrial tachycardia as triggered activity, abnormal automaticity, and reentry, despite the difficulties in differentiating between the former 2 mechanisms. Invasive studies have confirmed understanding of atrial tachycardia as a regular atrial activation generated by a pathologic mechanism from a small area spreading centrifugally. Because in a majority of cases atrial activation lasts less than the entire cycle length, there is a period of electrical inactivity, reflected on the ECG, as an isoelectric interval (**Fig. 8**). This remains the major, although not foolproof, differentiation criterion between focal atria tachycardia and macro-reentrant flutter. Rate of the tachycardia, the other time-honored differentiating criterion, has been shown highly unreliable

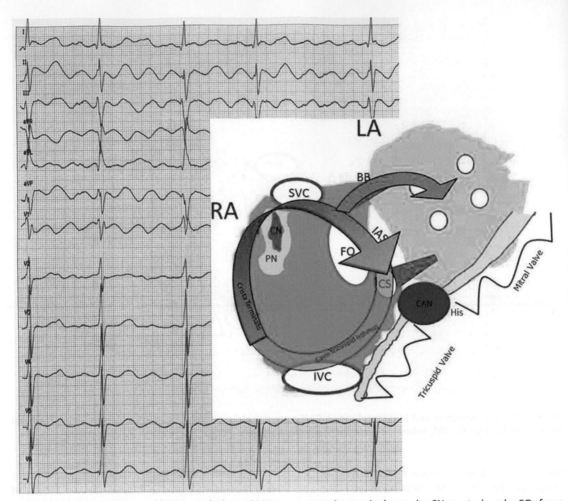

Fig. 7. CW AFL: anatomic and ECG correlations. CAN, compact atrioventricular node; CN, central node; FO, fossa ovalis; HIS, his bundle; IAS, interatrial septum; PN, perinodal zone; SN, sinus node.

because flutters and atrial tachycardias share a wide, overlapping range of cycle lengths. Extensive analysis of ECG tracings may identify other criteria, increasing atrial tachycardias' diagnostic accuracy. Among them, cycle-length variations are highly suggestive of an automatic mechanism (see **Fig. 8**). This is particularly true when the variability is associated with exercise or adrenergic stimulation or observed at the beginning (warming up) or the end (cooling down) of the arrhythmia. The origin of this tachycardia can be precisely identified observing the P-wave morphology (see Giuseppe Bagliani and colleagues' article, "P Wave and the Substrates of Arrhythmias Originating in the Atria," in this issue). Anatomic location and diagnostic ECG criteria of atrial tachycardia have been confirmed by numerous intracardiac mapping studies. Mapping has also shown the limitation of ECG for defining non–isthmus-dependent flutter and reentrant or

inappropriate sinus tachycardia or distinguishing between scars related to micro-reentry and macro-reentry.

Radiofrequency Ablation as Complicating Factor

The presence of atrial scars is not uncommon. Prosthetic material, ischemia, surgery, and long-standing hypertension, among other conditions, can generate islands of nonconductive tissue among normal myocardium. It is likely that in a majority of cases, these obstacles to propagation do not serve as a substrate for a macro-reentrant arrhythmias but the increased number of procedures causing atrial scars has increased their occurrences. Surgery, cryoablation, or radiofrequency ablation (RFA) of tissue around the pulmonary veins (PVs) and other specific left atrial (LA) locations during treatment of atrial

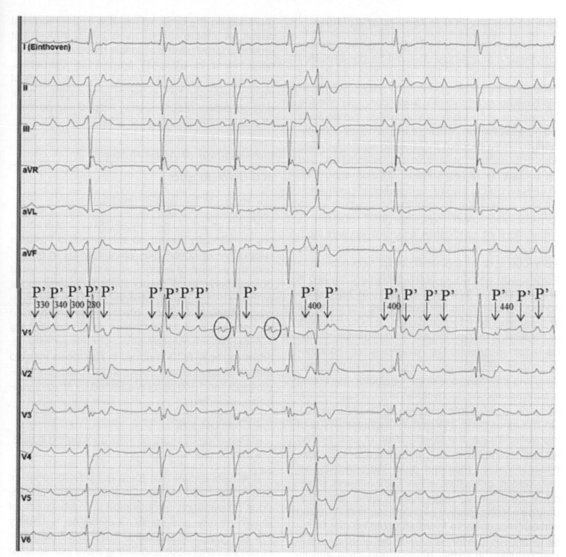

Fig. 8. Atrial tachycardia: recurrent episodes of atrial tachycardia (P′) and only isolated sinus atrial beats (*circles*). The P′-P′ cycle is variable (440–280 milliseconds).

fibrillation has made regular atrial arrhythmias originating in this cardiac chamber a common event. 3-D mapping has elucidated the variability of the reentrant circuits, the size of the scars, and their relationship to previous ablation but has not been as helpful in defining distinguishing ECG features of these arrhythmias. The uncertainty surrounding scar-related flutters depends on multiple factors. Obliteration of tissue reduces the overall voltage of the atrial recording, impeding a clear ECG analysis of the arrhythmia waveform. The extent of tissue obliteration can be inferred from the observation of sinus P wave. The more widespread the destruction, as in surgical maze or after multiple

extensive RFAs, the smaller the resultant P wave. Additionally, the creation of a large number of scar-related channels, bordered by electrophysiologically altered tissue, multiplies the possible paths of reentrant circuits, increasing the chance of concurrent arrhythmias. Finally, by destroying extensive regions of the LA, these procedures alter the intra-atrial and interatrial propagation of activation. ECG interpretation is based on knowledge of a certain pattern of electrical propagation. These atrial modifications, by introducing several unquantifiable changes to the progression of the activation wavefront, render the ECG interpretation of scar-related arrhythmias extremely problematic.

How to Use the ECG in the Era of Ablation

The interpretation of ECGs in present-day arrhythmia management does not have the primary role once enjoyed. The ease and safety of electrophysiological procedures have relegated this time-honored tool to a secondary role. Yet the information acquired by a knowledgeable analysis of a 12-lead tracing remains a fundamental complement to more modern therapeutic strategies. The likely mechanism of arrhythmia, its location, and the probability of response to ablation should be an integral part in the risk-versus-benefit evaluation guiding a decision to use this procedure or to consider alternative therapies. ECG analysis is today more complex than only a few years ago. There is more awareness of the limitations of this technique and of the relationship between wave morphology and origin of the tachycardias, and a large number of iatrogenic arrhythmias have been added to the ones naturally occurring. For clinicians approaching the interpretation of an ECG in the era of ablation, a few principles, reviewed later, should be kept in mind. The diagnosis of isthmus-dependent AFL, the site of origin of atrial tachycardias, and the relevance of the isoelectric line during a supraventricular tachycardia are concepts firmly ensconced in the interpretation of the ECG tracing. On the other hand, the limited diagnostic value of tachycardia rate, the identification of scar-related flutters' reentrant circuit, and the distinction between focal or reentrant atrial tachycardias are new added difficulties. Even ECG features previously considered diagnostic of atrial fibrillation may be not as definitive as once assumed. A tracing without recognizable P waves could be due to the simultaneous presence of multiple organized flutters resulting in highly disorganized atrial activity indistinguishable from atrial fibrillation. Furthermore, knowledge of a patient's previous ablations and observation of the alterations induced on the sinus P wave by previous procedures should become a fundamental part of the ECG evaluation of every atrial arrhythmia. These limitations, notwithstanding the ratio of cost versus information gathered, continues to makes a 12-lead ECG the most common test in clinical cardiac practice. Future studies continuing to compare intracardiac and ECG recordings will provide an opportunities to clarify the features of these complex arrhythmias and attain more definitive diagnostic criteria.

ATRIAL FLUTTER
Introduction

AFL is a macro-reentrant atrial tachycardia. This definition separates micro-reentries from macro-reentries on the basis of the size of the reentrant circuit. A macro-reentry is a circus movement around a large central obstacle measuring several centimeters in at least one of its diameters. Although, as discussed previously, the nature of the obstacle can be functional or fixed, this article only considers macro-reentry around a large fixed obstacle either anatomic or scar.

Classification of Atrial Flutter

ECG characteristics

- Rate and features of atrial activation

The ECG criteria to classify AFL in clinical practice are traditionally based on the rate and features supportive of continuous atrial activity. In reality, with the advent of endocavitary mapping, several observations have demonstrated the limitations of the ECG diagnosis. Mapping and electrophysiology studies, however, are the gold standard in the diagnosis of AFL; 12-lead ECG remains the initial approach to the diagnosis of this arrhythmia. From multiple ECG reports, is has been learned that atrial rate (usually between 240 beats per minute [bpm] and 340 bpm) is affected by several variables, including

- Chamber size
- Presence of scars or slow conducting tissue
- Medications

It is also known that there is no fixed range of rates diagnostic of AFL. On the contrary, continuous propagation of activation is the hallmark of macro-reentry and its ECG evidence is usually the key diagnostic feature. The ECG tracing inscribes a continuous undulating wave with specific characteristics without an isoelectric line (see **Figs. 1**, **6**, and **7**). Studies correlating ECG and intracavitary recordings of atrial activation have allowed understanding the genesis of the ECG waveforms in AFL. Based on these observations, it is possible to reconstruct, fairly precisely, the path followed by the macro-reentrant tachycardias by ECG analysis and to recognize characteristic patterns associated with specific reentrant paths.

Isthmus-dependent and non–isthmus-dependent atrial flutter

The classification of AFL is based on well-defined ECG criteria that reflect the role played by the isthmus between the tricuspid valve and the inferior vena cava (IVC) in the maintenance of the macro-reentry (see **Figs. 6** and **7**). In the so-called isthmus-dependent flutter, also referred as typical or type I, this structure is a necessary part of the reentrant circuit. In atypical flutter or type II (see **Fig. 5**), also called non–isthmus-dependent, the circus movement is confined by other anatomic structures and the function of the isthmus is secondary. In isthmus-dependent flutter, the right atrium (RA) is activated by a waveform exiting the isthmus and propagating to the rest of the atria in a predictable fashion with a stable velocity of conduction. Because the wavefront rotates around the tricuspid valve, for an observer hypothetically looking at the valve from the apex of the right ventricle, 2 possible activation directions are possible: CW or CCW (see **Figs. 6** and **7**). Either of the 2 rotations generates a tracing with standard features and minor variations. On the other hand, atypical AFL, as the name implies, is a macro-reentry bound by less predictable barriers, contained either within the LA or RA, with a propagation path that is often difficult to reconstruct by analysis based solely on ECG tracings (see **Fig. 5**). Although some features suggest the chamber of origin and the overall direction of the wavefront, the complete reconstruction of this arrhythmia requires endocardial mapping and 3-D reconstruction.

Isthmus Dependent Atrial Flutter or Typical Atrial Flutter

Counterclockwise flutter

The most common and most recognizable feature of typical CCW flutter on ECG is the presence of sawtooth waves in the inferior leads without a clear return to baseline. A close look at the components of the waves in these derivations shows a positive wave followed by a slowly descending plateau and a rapid negative deflection (see **Fig. 1**; **Fig. 9**). It is expected that the inferior leads provide a majority of information for the genesis of the depolarization vectors but complementary observation can be gathered by the analysis of waveforms in leads V1, V6, I, and aVL.[1–4] In general, in both types of isthmus-dependent flutter, the overall morphology of the F waves is determined by LA activation, and any change in the pattern of activation of this chamber leads to major ECG variations.

Beginning with the analysis of the stereotypical sawtooth pattern, the first component, always inferior in the inferior leads, reflects the activation of the RA septum and posterior LA wall (see **Fig. 9**). The depolarizing wavefront reaches the inferior septal

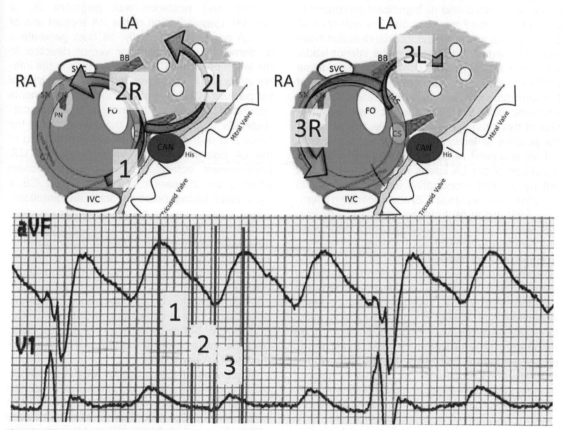

Fig. 9. CCW, isthmus-dependent AFL. The sequences of activation of the atria and the corresponding ECG sawtooth pattern (see text for further details). CAN, compact atrioventricular node; CN, central node; FO, fossa ovalis; HIS, his bundle; IAS, interatrial septum; PN, perinodal zone; SN, sinus node.

wall, exiting the cavotricuspid isthmus (CVI) (segment 1 of **Fig. 9**), and ascends along the septum and posteriorly toward the crista terminalis (CT) (segment 2R of **Fig. 9**). Invading the coronary sinus, the activation begins the depolarization of the LA directed initially caudocranially, posteroanteriorly, and toward the left (segment 2L of **Fig. 9**). The LA also is activated by a second depolarizing wave of opposite polarity when the septal propagation reaches the Bachmann bundle (BB) located at the septal apex (segment 3L of **Fig. 9**). Although anteriorly the RA propagation advances along the tricuspid valve toward the lateral wall (segment 3R of **Fig. 9**), the progression of the posterior wavefront is blocked by the CT and forced superiorly in the space between the superior vena cava (SVC) and the CT. From this space, it turns around and proceeds inferiorly along the anterior wall. The CT separates these 2 wavefronts, preventing early short circuiting and extinction of the activation in the anterior wall as they proceed in opposite directions. In reality, a small degree of fusion of these wavefronts occurs in the presence of conduction gaps in the CT; however, the overall vector of activation, in a great majority of cases, remains unchanged and no significant morphologic alterations of the F waves occur. The activation of the RA lateral wall in a caudocranial direction interrupts the negative deflection in the inferior leads, inscribing a short positive component in the same ECG derivatives. Activation of the LA proceeds at the same time with, in a majority of cases, a posteroanterior vector directed to the left. The depolarization of this chamber is responsible, therefore, for the positive deflection in V1 (posteroanterior activation) and positive deflections in I and aVL. The activation of the LA lateral wall is mostly carried out by the fast propagating wavefront emerging from the coronary sinus (CS) and ascending inferosuperiorly and away from the most lateral precordial leads. This vector consequently determines the negative polarity of V6 observed in the great majority of CCW flutter.

From the lateral wall, the activation is forced by the eustachian ridge into CVI. The amount of tissue depolarizing in normal conditions during this stage is minimal and, having completed LA activation, there is no other wavefront of activity to be recorded. The corresponding ECG deflection is not an isoelectric line but a flat line with inferior tilt resembling a plateau. The normal duration of the isthmus activation is approximately 100 milliseconds to 140 milliseconds; a longer extent suggests a slowing of conduction velocity as it is observed after incomplete isthmus ablations or undetermined scarring of this anatomic region (**Fig. 10**). The shorter the isthmus conduction, the

more likely a continuous undulating activity is present in the ECG; the longer the conduction, the more likely a complete return to baseline is observed.

Clockwise flutter

Less commonly, the rotation of the arrhythmia proceeds in CW direction around the tricuspid valve. The arrhythmia boundaries are the same but the propagation wavefront exits the isthmus at its free wall ending, thereby engaging the other segments of the RA in a opposite direction (**Fig. 11**). The function of the CT is again to ensure that the major anteriorly propagating wave is not short circuited by the superiorly directed propagation with termination of the flutter. The overall polarity of the F wave is initially negative in the inferior leads, as the wavefront ascends toward the SVC on the free wall (segment 1 of **Fig. 11**) before turning rightward along the anterior wall toward the septum. The septum is activated next in a craniocaudal direction (segment 2R of **Fig. 11**) whereas the BB is invaded earlier. This generates an activation propagating in the LA from the superoanterior region, proceeding inferiorly along the anterior and posterior wall (segment 2L of **Fig. 11**). Depolarization of the RA septum and of the LA occurs concurrently; as both generate a predominantly superoinferior vector directed to the left, a positive ECG deflection both in the inferior leads and in V6 is inscribed. A close analysis of the positive ECG wave often shows 2 components separated by a notch. The timing of the notch corresponds to the arrival of the wavefront at the lower end of the septum and to the beginning of the LA posterior wall activation along the CS. Concomitant activation of the subeustachian isthmus and concentric activation of the CS is meanwhile taking place in opposite directions. These 2 simultaneous biatrial wavefronts moving in opposite directions do not cancel each other but create an interaction between their respective electromotive forces and generate a distinct dipolar surface on body map distribution and a notch on 12-lead ECG.

CVI activation occurs concomitantly with LA depolarization. As a consequence, in the 12-lead ECG of CW flutter there is no plateau recorded because this portion of the F wave registers the dominant LA activation.

Differences in the activation of this chamber, determined by variable dominance of 1 or the other of the 2 LA wavefronts, determine the last portion of the F wave. This is seen particularly with leads more obviously affected by anteroposterior (V1) or lateral (aVL, I, or V6) vectors. In the majority of cases, the main deflection is positive

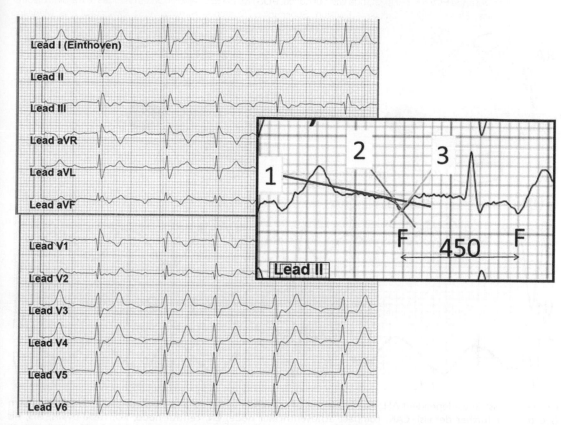

Fig. 10. Slow CCW AFL (in patient taking amiodarone). The isthmus-dependent conduction (*red line*) is prolonged. The remainder of right and left atrial activation (Blue and Green lines) is unchanged.

in V6 and negative in V1, suggestive of a predominant activation spreading from the BB and directed anterior to posterior and leftward.

Left atrial activation in typical atrial flutter

In typical AFL, the LA is a bystander chamber, passively activated and not necessary to maintain this arrhythmia. Nevertheless, several animal and human studies have shown that the activation of this chamber mostly determines the wave polarity in the 12-lead ECG. There are 2 dominant interatrial pathways, BB and CS (see **Figs. 6**, **7**, **9**, and **11**). The former is, in normal circumstances, the main interatrial connection. It is situated in the anterior roof of the LA and generates a propagation directed superoinferiorly from the anterior toward the posterior LA wall. The latter pathway, situated inferiorly and posteriorly, produces a wavefront directed in the opposite direction. The resultant LA depolarizing wave in AFL, therefore, reflects a variable degree of fusion between these 2 opposite activations (see **Figs. 9** and **11**). The polarity of the main ECG vectors depends on the balance between these 2 waves, which is related to the sequence of activation and the

conduction velocity along these 2 interatrial connections. The CS os is activated, in normal atria, approximately 44 milliseconds before the BB region in CCW flutter (see **Figs. 9**) and 52 milliseconds after the BB region in CW flutter (see **Fig. 11**). In CCW flutter (see **Fig. 9**; **Fig. 12**), the earliest activation proceeds caudocranially from the CS and for 44 milliseconds is unopposed inscribing characteristic inferior negative F waves. On the contrary, in CW flutter, the BB is engaged first, generating an opposite direction of activation and positive F waves in the same leads (see **Figs. 11** and **12**). V1 is also a powerful discriminator between the 2 types of AFL: positive in CCW reflecting a posteroanterior direction of activation and negative in CW, where the wavefront mostly propagates in the opposite direction. The terminal segment of the F wave also represents a combination of different LA and RA wavefronts. In CW, the negative deflection is the result of concordant activations of the lateral wall of both atria. These portions of the chambers are both depolarized in an inferior-superior direction by the CS wavefront in the LA and by the emergence of the isthmus propagation wave in the RA. In

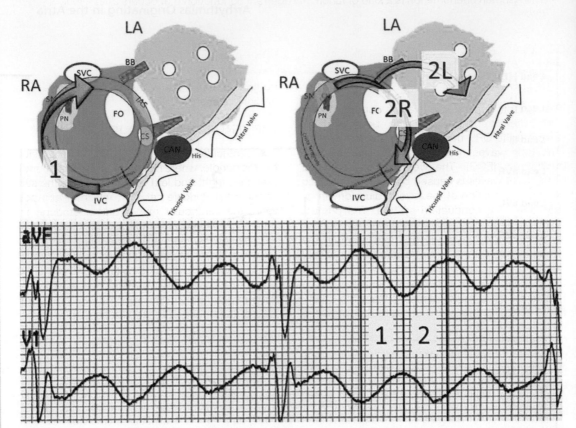

Fig. 11. CW, isthmus-dependent AFL. The sequences of activation of the atria and the corresponding ECG pattern (see text for further details). CAN, compact atrioventricular node; CN, central node; FO, fossa ovalis; HIS, his bundle; IAS, interatrial septum; PN, perinodal zone; SN, sinus node.

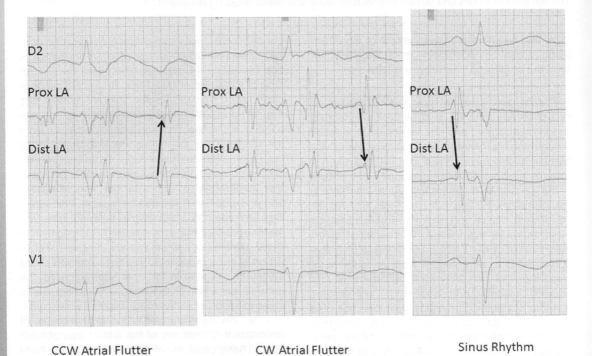

Fig. 12. LA activation recorded by esophageal leads during CCW and CW Atrial Flutter and Sinus Rhythm. The arrows indicate the direction of LA activation. The activation is caudocranial in CCW, from distal (Dist) to proximal (Prox) LA, and the opposite in CW. The activation in Sinus Rhythm is similar to CW Atrial Flutter.

CCW, the RA wavefront descending from the superior aspect of the free wall is unopposed because the depolarization of the LA is mostly concluded. The resultant ECG deflection is, therefore, positive.

In summary, the LA can be considered a modulator of the morphology of the surface ECG in AFL. This is particularly true of CW flutter, where the depolarization of this chamber occurs mostly during plateau depolarization and is, therefore, unopposed by RA-generated vectors. In this type of flutter, the contribution of the 2 interatrial connections is likely to affect the ECG configuration of the flutter more than in CCW.

Slowing or block of conduction of the CS or BB route shifts the balance of LA activation with different degrees of wavefront fusion, but it is difficult to estimate, during sinus rhythm or during the arrhythmia, the degree of conduction delays or blocks in these 2 pathways. Polarity reversal of inferior waves in CCW AFL after CS block has been reported,[5] demonstrating the dependence of F-wave morphology on the predominant path of LA activation. Furthermore, there is evidence that LA enlargement or heart disease influence the right to left propagation during typical AFL-inducing unpredictable changes in F-wave morphology.[6] It is also important to stress that multiple variations exist in the balance of activation between these 2 depolarizing wavefronts, and it is likely that subtle

variations of dominance are undetected by the 12-lead ECG. Variations in the ECG morphology of isthmus-dependent flutter are important and they are the subject of the next article.

ECG variants of isthmus-dependent flutter

What has been described so far is the typical progression of an activation wave along a well-established flutter circuit. This results in the stereotypical ECG appearance, which is recognized as CCW or CW flutter. In reality, several variations exist and a typical appearance of either flutter is present only in approximately 30% of the cases.[6] For CCW flutter, the necessary diagnostic feature is the negative sawtooth morphology in the inferior leads accompanied by a small terminal positive deflection. Changes in the ratio of these 2 components are common (**Figs. 13** and **14**) and include a monophasic negative F wave, a negative dominant F wave with a small terminal positive wave, and a predominantly positive F wave with a small initial negative component. The negative component is, as discussed previously, determined by the simultaneous caudocranial activation of the septum and of the LA, where the depolarization begins from the CS. Any variation in this sequence can induce a large range of ECG changes from subtle to considerable. Both the lower and the higher interatrial connections can develop variable degrees of conduction block, changing the balance of LA

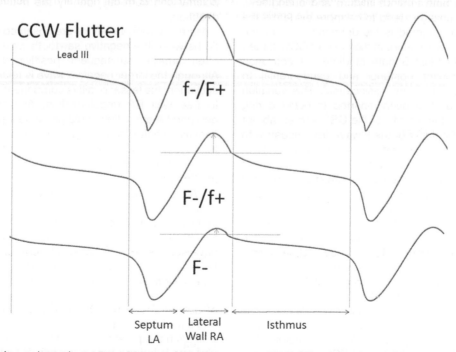

Fig. 13. Isthmus-dependent AFL variants: a schematic representation of the different morphology of sawtooth F wave in the inferior leads. The ratio between the negative and the final positive deflection varies from a completely negative to a mostly positive deflection (see text for further details).

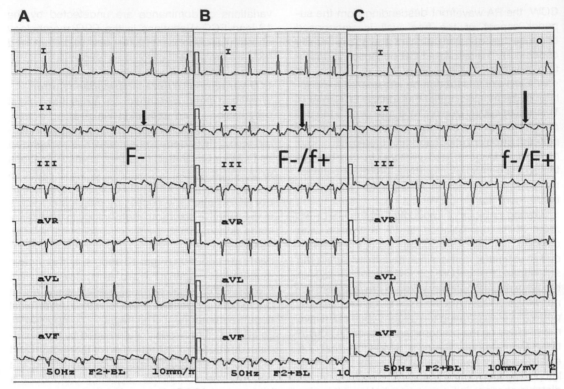

Fig. 14. Isthmus-dependent AFL variants: Different ratios between the negative and the final positive atrial deflection; the positive terminal component progressively increases from A to C (*arrows*); see text for further details.

activation both in sinus rhythm and during AFL. The ECG changes tend to be more evident if the connection affected is the dominant one for the type of flutter rotation. In the case of CCW flutter, a block in the CS path modifies LA activation from dominant posterior and caudocranial to mostly superior and craniocaudal. This variation in activation has been reported to occur during ablation in the vicinity of the CS[7] with an abrupt change of polarity of the F wave from negative to positive without alterations in cycle length or RA activation sequence. Mapping of the CS wavefront demonstrated a change of activation sequence explaining the alterations of F wave polarity. These findings strongly suggest that LA activation converted from a predominant caudocranial depolarization from the CS to a superoinferior activation proceeding from BB. These observations occurred, as discussed previously, both spontaneously[5] or as a consequence of RFA.[7]

The ECG reflects the altered activation of the LA with reversal of waveform polarity in lead I in the inferior leads and in V6. Leads V1 and aVL remained mostly positive. After the modification of LA activation, the overall ECG appearance is more consistent with CW flutter despite an unchanged CCW rotation. Observing V1 and aVL

polarity can correctly identify the macro-reentry direction.

More common variations are observed in the ratio between the negative sawtooth wave and the often smaller subsequent positive deflection. Although the larger negative wave is related to LA activation, the lesser positive component is related to free wall RA depolarization. Any condition-delaying LA activation could generate a persisting negative vector counterbalancing the one from the RA. The result could be a dominant negative F wave with small or no positive component. On the contrary, extensive left posterior wall ablation for AF can lead to substantial loss of this wall voltage. In this case, the caudocranial activation of the RA free wall results in a more dominant positive component on the ECG.[8] Some investigators have suggested a possible relationship between the shape of the RA and the dominance of the positive deflection. The more elongated the RA, the longer the free wall generating a longitudinal vector of depolarization with higher voltage amplitudes and a more marked positive deflection.[9]

In a small subset of patients with CCW, the regular rate is interrupted by periods of faster tachycardia with subtle ECG changes, such as loss of the terminal positive deflection of the flutter in the inferior leads. One of the possible causes of this phenomenon is the emergence of an activation front skirting the posterior wall of the IVC, breaking through at the level of the inferior RA and reentering the isthmus at that level.[10] In this case, the circuit rotates around the IVC but remains isthmus dependent. The major characteristics of this flutter are a shorter different path, hence the faster rate, and the depolarization of the lateral wall in a caudocranial path opposite to the direction of typical CCW flutter. The wavefront ascends the lateral wall, colliding with the wavefront proceeding from the SVC. The resultant vector is a combination of 2 small opposite ones and on the ECG it is manifested by a loss of the positive terminal deflection.

Flutter sustained by CW rotation around the tricuspid valve is far less common than the opposite counterpart and, therefore, fewer detailed observations of ECG variability during this arrhythmia are available. ECG morphology of CW mostly represents LA activation, which occurs in great part during CVI depolarization and is, therefore, unopposed by RA-generated electrical vectors. A shift in LA activation pattern from craniocaudal to inferosuperior has seldom been reported to occur spontaneously during electrophysiologic studies without change in RA activation or cycle length.[10]

Non Isthmus Dependent Atrial Flutter

Upper loop reentry
A rare form of nonisthmus flutter is called upper loop reentry.[11] This is not a well-defined entity but rather a definition encompassing several arrhythmias sharing some common features. All seem to be macro-reentry non–isthmus-dependent tachycardias, mostly occurring during typical flutter and due to some anomalies of the CT. This anatomic structure demonstrates variable conduction block, either related to its fiber arrangement or to its response to higher rate of stimulation. Gaps in the line of block or areas of inhomogeneous conduction can favor, during typical flutter, formation of different smaller circuits incorporating the CT as the most important component. In one of the reported arrhythmias, the circuit can be considered a variation of typical flutter, most commonly CW. In this case, the wavefront of activation shifts from its usual path to a circuit around the SVC rotating around this vein through a small gap in the CT. In this case, the crista provides, thanks to its inhomogeneous conduction properties, a slow conduction area that allows the perpetuation of a circus movement around the SVC.

Activation of the LA, after the exit of the wavefront from the gap in the upper CT, proceeds

as in typical CW flutter, whereas in the RA, 2 wavefronts are generated colliding most often just outside the isthmus. The ECG morphology is, therefore, often similar to CW flutter.[11,12]

Another better documented non–isthmus-dependent upper loop reentry rotates around the entire CT, exiting at 2 gaps in this line of block: at the upper level of the SVC and at the inferior RA wall in front of the isthmus. The overall ECG appearance is consistent with CW flutter, because the upper wavefront exiting the loop is in close vicinity of the origin of the BB; the LA, therefore, is activated as in CW flutter.[11] Nevertheless it is important to differentiate between typical CW flutter and this more unusual CT circuit, because this information can determine the RFA approach. An ECG finding that may help differentiate between these 2 flutters is the different appearance of lead I. In this upper loop reentry, the F wave is often negative or isoelectric with amplitude less than or equal to 0.07 mV. On the contrary, in isthmus-dependent CW flutter, the same lead has a clear positive deflection. This ECG change could be explained by different timing of activation of the RA free wall in these 2 macro-reentries.[13] In CW flutter, the RA wall is activated first whereas in upper loop reentry the RA wall is activated at the same time as the LA. This generates 2 vectors, with opposite direction and parallel to the axis of lead I.

Scar-related flutters
As previously defined, macro-reentry circuit requires a stable reentrant path limited by anatomic and or acquired boundaries. An essential part of the circuit is a segment of tissue, called an isthmus, with slow conduction properties delimited by areas of nonconduction. Although this may be a simplified model, it is useful in explaining the initiation and maintenance of this arrhythmia and the ECG findings associated with it. The CVI serves, as discussed previously, as the critical link of the so-called typical flutters. Other areas of slow conductions and new boundaries can be produced in either atria by surgical or catheter-based procedures creating scars, adding prosthetic material, or remodeling of these chambers due to volume, pressure overload, or long-standing atrial arrhythmias. The addition of proarrhythmic substrate to cardiac chambers already anatomically predisposed to or rhythmias creates a large number of macro-reentries generically referred to as scar-related tachycardias or atypical flutters.

The are many variables determining the ECG features of scar-related flutters, including, among others, anatomic location of the scar, direction of rotation of the reentry, number of active reentrant paths, effects of antiarrhythmic drugs, volume of the chamber, role of the CVI, and the extent of atrial myocyte loss. It is, therefore, not surprising that, contrary to isthmus-dependent flutters, the electrographic manifestations of these arrhythmias are neither fully understood nor standardized.

Right atrium scar-related atrial flutter

A majority of RA atypical flutters are related to previous surgical procedures where this chamber is accessed by a lateral atriotomy or when large SVC- IVC incisions are created to introduce extracorporeal circulation cannulas or when a surgical patch is sutured on the septum to correct atrial septal defects. Other scars can develop in nonsurgical patients; in these cases, their etiology is far more speculative as in patients with no history of CV disease.

3-D mapping has greatly clarified the numerous anatomic locations of the reentrant pathways in this flutters but, in view of the uniqueness of each arrhythmia, it has not provided standardized ECG criteria to interpret them.

Nevertheless, some generalized observations can be made to help in the diagnosis of the macro-reentry.

In a great majority of these arrhythmias, the CVI is involved in the reentry, either as the sole mechanism or in combination with another concurrent arrhythmia.[14] CW rotation around the tricuspid valve is observed far more often in the presence of surgically manipulated atria than in virgin chambers. It is unclear why this is the case and it can only be speculated that, at least in some cases, the flutter is CCW with a reversed LA activation, as discussed previously. In this case, observation of a positive lead V1 should clarify the issue. It is also possible that alterations in the usual anatomic boundaries force the wavefront reentry in a CW direction. The more extensive the surgery, the slower the rate of the arrhythmia. Furthermore, a longer conduction across an isolated isthmus leads to a period of low or no electrical potential and the recording of an isoelectric line. Often the implicated area is a region of scarred tissue where the wavefront propagates very slowly due to abnormal conduction. A clear isoelectric line is frequently observed in patients with a septal patch and, in 1 report, it seemed diagnostic of double-loop reentry involving a lateral wall scar and the CVI. On the contrary, conduction through an enlarged chamber with a great deal of myopathic tissue results in a slow continuous electrical activity of low but appreciable voltage. An undulating, regular waveform of low voltage in all leads is at

times observed, making it difficult to obtain detailed observations, save for the wave polarity. Finally, some studies have suggested that in situations where the ECG is difficult to interpret, a completely negative lead V1 represents a reliable marker of RA origin of the flutter. On the contrary, a completely positive or biphasic appearance of this lead with initial positive deflection is far more consistent with LA flutters. There are no studies in the literature directly correlating the morphology of this lead with endocavitary biatrial activation to explain the mechanism of this observation. This association is, therefore, mostly based on empiric clinical observations.

Left atrial scar-related atrial flutter

Although the RA is anatomically predisposed to develop flutter, the LA has no strategically located boundaries that can easily be transformed in reentrant pathways. AFL in normal LA is almost unknown. On the other hand, development of conduction blocks or areas of slow propagation, either due to iatrogenic interventions or myopathic processes, can easily transform this chamber in the receptacle of macroreentry arrhythmias. After the exponential increase in surgical or catheter-based procedures developed for the treatment of AF, there has been an equally large number of reports of atypical LA flutters. The great majority of these reports illustrate macro-reentrant or micro-reentrant arrhythmias dependent on scars, most commonly produced during pulmonary veins (PVs) isolation or after the creation of ablation lines in surgical or catheter-based maze-type procedures. Microreentry atrial tachycardia is a tachycardia with spread of activation from a focal point and a mechanism consistent with a very small reentrant circuit. The diagnosis of this arrhythmia requires evaluation of the principles of reentry during electrophysiology study, because it is, at times, difficult to distinguish it with ECG from a macroreentry tachycardia. In general, the ECG features of a microreentry P-wave morphology are similar to those of premature beats or pace-maps of PVs previously described (see Giuseppe Bagliani and colleagues' article, "P Wave and the Substrates of Arrhythmias Originating in the Atria," in this issue).[15] On the contrary, scar-related macroreentrant flutters present with several variable morphologies depending, as discussed previously, on multiple determinants. In general, the more extensive the scarring induced by the procedure, the least predictable the F-wave morphology. The most common reentrant pathways involve a perimitral circuit around the mitral valve (MV) or around scars encircling left, right, or all PVs. The addition of linear ablations and more extensive scarring induced by substrate modification adds a considerable uncertainty to the ECG interpretation of these arrhythmias. Furthermore, there are no detailed studies relating the morphology of the F wave of these arrhythmias to the progression of the wavefronts in the LA, preventing a reconstruction of the arrhythmia pathway from ECG analysis. Several studies have tried to collect sufficient data to allow an observer to identify the chamber of origin of the arrhythmia and differentiate perimetral MV flutters from arrhythmias rotating around other ablation-induced obstacles. Despite that no specific ECG pattern predicts accurately any of the commonest circuits, some generalizations are possible. The perimetral MV flutter is the arrhythmia that most lends itself to ECG standardization.[16] The perimeter around the MV is normally unable to sustain AFL, unless other nonanatomic boundaries are created to force the reentrant path along the valve annulus. This perimetral flutter is not an uncommon complication after ablations for AF or in the presence of myopathic scars in the anterior or posterior wall of the LA. The direction of rotation around the valve dictates the main ECG features of this arrhythmia with a positive F wave both in the inferior leads and V1 in CCW flutter. The opposite inferior lead morphology was observed in CW direction of reentry, but V1 remained positive. V1 in both flutters seems broad and often double humped, and some investigators have suggested that the broader this wave, the more likely the circuit is perimetral MV. Other leads may present more variations and they seem diagnostically less useful. This arrhythmia was never observed in multiple reports to have an isoelectric line separating the F waves.

How to Read a Flutter ECG

An arrhythmia with an ECG appearance of a regular monomorphic, highly reproducible, continuously undulating wave is defined as AFL. These features are not always present in every macro-reentrant tachycardia. In particular, rate is highly nonspecific for AFL and at times, instead of a continuous line, this arrhythmia exhibits the presence of an isoelectric line[a] between F waves.

When confronted with a 12-lead ECG of an AFL, the first and possibly most important determination is to understand the atrial chamber of origin

and if originating in the RA, whether the flutter is isthmus dependent.

From the authors' previous analysis, typical flutter is diagnosed when some stereotypical features are present:

1. A continuous wave is much more likely to be present than an isoelectric line.
2. In CCW, the F wave recorded in the inferior leads should include a sawtooth component followed by a descending plateau and a positive deflection. In particular, the small positive deflection, when present, is highly specific for typical CCW flutter. The plateau, of characteristic descending slope, should not last more than 120 milliseconds to 140 milliseconds. Notching of the descending and ascending branches of the sawtooth is uncommon and it should direct the diagnosis toward a different mechanism or a combination of mechanisms (ie, double-loop flutters). V1 is almost always completely positive or biphasic with a positive-negative deflection. V6 is also always negative and aVR is a mirror image of the inferior leads with a biphasic positive-negative wave.
3. In CW flutter, the inferior leads record a positive wave with a small notch interrupting the ascending branch approximately half way. Again, the presence of the small notch and its location are highly specific for this type of flutter. V1 and aVR are predominantly negative and V6 positive.

The more the features of the observed tracing match this pattern, the more likely it is that the macro-reentry is isthmus dependent. Making a correct diagnosis of typical AFL in the presence of potential confounding factors is difficult. In general, any alteration of interatrial connections or substantial loss of LA mass alters the ECG appearance of typical flutter often beyond recognition.

In general, if the LA has been instrumented by an ablative procedure—catheter, balloon, or surgically based—the resultant arrhythmia, either micro-reentrant or macro-reentrant, is far more likely to originate from this chamber. Nevertheless, isthmus-dependent flutter in patients without a previous ablation of the CTI represents approximately 30% of post-AF ablation recurrences. Ablative procedures can markedly decrease LA viable tissue and modify interatrial connections, altering the ECG presentation of

---

[a]An isoelectric line is defined as line returning to baseline present in all 12 lead ECG with a duration empirically defined of at least 80 milliseconds. The low voltage recorded corresponds to the period without electrical activity (in focal tachycardia) or the time of propagation of the wavefront through an area of low voltage (as in diseased cells or a slow conducting isthmus in a reentry circuit).

isthmus-dependent flutter. Not infrequently, CCW flutter after LA ablation for AF presents with inferior positive F waves and positive V1 despite preserved interatrial connections.[16] The ECG appearance is possibly related to the extensive ablation of the posterior LA wall. The loss of tissue decreases the magnitude of the depolarizing caudocranial vector of this wall and leaves the anterior wall craniocaudal activation mostly unopposed. Review of the P wave in sinus rhythm (SR) can yield useful information helping in the interpretation of arrhythmias. Marked sinus P waves changes are observed, for example, after maze procedure for AF. This is an open heart procedure performed mostly concomitantly with other cardiovascular surgeries where the surgeon encircles, using a radiofrequency probe, every PV and performs several linear ablations in both atria. The modification of the atrial tissue is profound and results in sinus P waves that are usually of less than 0.1 mV voltage in every lead, with frequent loss of the negative component in V1 and a dominant positive morphology in all inferior and precordial leads. Most of the arrhythmias after this procedure are macro-reentry, including, in up to one-third of the cases, isthmus-dependent flutters. In every maze-related arrhythmia the ECG is highly atypical, probably because of the extensive LA debulking, and often even typical flutter cannot be identified correctly.

In summary, despite the increasingly dominant role assumed by invasive procedures in the treatment of arrhythmias, ECG analysis remains an important diagnostic tool in the identification of the mechanism of tachycardias. The correct identification of the circuit of reentry and the chamber of origin can substantially help in the preparation for the arrhythmia ablation.

More correlations between mapping of the endocavitary path of reentry with the resultant ECG manifestations are needed to be able to interpret correctly the tracings of scar-related arrhythmias. Following the example of previous researchers, who splendidly clarified the mechanism of typical flutter, it behooves the new generation of invasive electrophysiologists to continue the study of these arrhythmias bridging the gap between endocavitary and surface ECG findings.

ATRIAL TACHYCARDIAS

Atrial tachycardias originate in sites different from sinus node, and are characterized by a non-physiological behavior (**Fig. 15**).

The relationship between P and QRS depends on the tachycardia rate and on the atrioventricular node (AVN) capability to conduct all or some atrial depolarization. If the rate of the tachycardia is faster than the depolarization properties of the AVN, this structure blocks some of the atrial activations, inducing a P/QRS ratio greater than 1 (**Fig. 16**). Additionally, the extreme variability of the R-R intervals can lead to an erroneous diagnosis of AF (**Fig. 17**).

Atrioventricular conduction can be modified by drugs or by an increasing vagal tone independently from the tachycardia rate. This finding is useful in differentiating atrial from junctional or accessory pathway-mediated tachycardias, where the AVN is an integral part of the circuit and P and QRS are persistently associated.

Reentry and enhanced automatic drive are the mechanisms of atrial tachycardias. Sinus node reentry and scar-related tachycardias are part of the first group; automatic and multifocal atrial tachycardias belong to the second.

Automatic Atrial Tachycardia

The automatic atrial tachycardia arrhythmia (see **Fig. 15**), due to enhanced automatism, is characterized, like all other automatic tachycardias, by a rate acceleration (warming up) at the onset and a rate decrease (cooling down) just before the end of the arrhythmia. Additionally, rate is often variable during the course of the arrhythmia.

The P-wave morphology of atrial tachycardia differs from sinus P wave. Its analysis allows anatomic localization of the arrhythmia origin, as discussed previously for ectopic atrial beats (see Giuseppe Bagliani and colleagues' article, "P Wave and the Substrates of Arrhythmias Originating in the Atria," in this issue). The atrial tachycardia rate can reach 200 bpm with fusion of the P wave in the preceding T wave (P/T phenomenon) (see **Fig. 16**). The P-Q interval during this arrhythmia can vary but is often longer than in normal sinus rhythm. This can be due to propagation of the ectopic impulse along normal working myocardium and to a decremental response of the AVN to faster rates (see **Fig. 16**).

Multifocal atrial tachycardia is due to increased spontaneous automaticity of multiple atrial foci (**Fig. 18**). ECG diagnosis is based on the identification of at least 3 distinct P-wave morphologies. Multifocal atrial tachycardia is usually observed in patients with chronic obstructive lung disease treated with aminophylline and in patients with congestive heart failure; this arrhythmia often degenerates into AF.

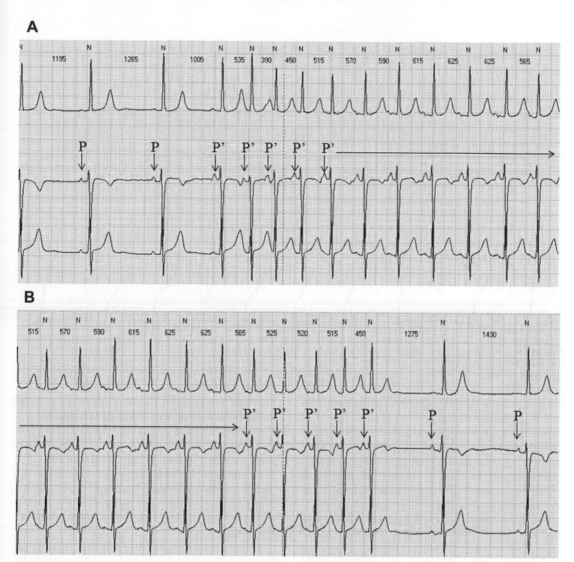

Fig. 15. Paroxysmal atrial tachycardia (hyperautomatic): after 2 sinus beats (*P*) a paroxysm of atrial tachycardia (*P'*) starts (*A*) and ends (*B*). The P'–P' varies significantly during the paroxysm.

Sinus Node Reentry

Sinus node reentry and scar-related tachycardia are both atrial arrhythmias due to reentry. As in any other reentrant arrhythmia, the circuit of sinus node reentry requires an area of slow conduction. This region is localized at the level of the sinoatrial connection, hence the designation sinus node reentry tachycardias (**Fig. 19**). The rate of this arrhythmia is not high, varying between 130 bpm and 180 bpm. The P-wave morphology is similar to the sinus wave because both originate in the same anatomic region, making the distinction between sinus tachycardia and sinus node reentry tachycardia difficult. One important

distinguishing feature is the mode of initiation of these arrhythmias: progressive in sinus tachycardia, sudden and often beginning with a premature atrial beat in sinus node reentry tachycardia.

Scar-Related Atrial Tachycardia

As previously discussed in the article of AFL, a focal tachycardia can originate from a small micro-reentrant circuit. Although all the principles of reentry apply to this diminutive reentrant path, the ECG features of this arrhythmia are consistent with focal tachycardia. Nevertheless, there are no specific features diagnostic of this tachycardia. As discussed previously, even rate and presence

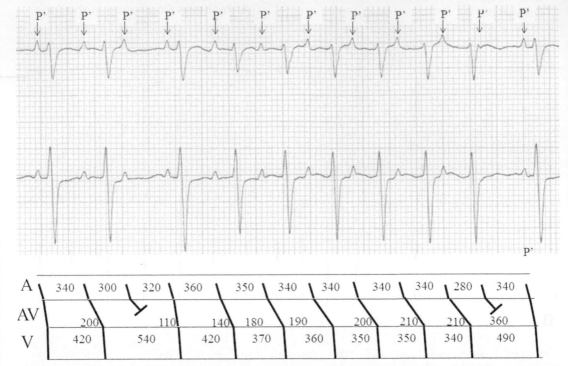

A	340	300	320	360	350	340	340	340	340	280	340
AV	200		110	140	180	190	200	210	210	360
V	420	540		420	370	360	350	350	340	490

Fig. 16. Atrial tachycardia: a detail of **Fig. 3** shows an atrial tachycardia (average P'–P' = 340 milliseconds); occasional P'–P' shortenings (300 and 280 milliseconds) are associated with atrioventricular conduction 2: 1 (Wenckebach-like). Often, P wave is inserted in the T wave of the previous beat (the P/T phenomenon). A, atrium; AV, atrio-ventricular junction; V, ventricle.

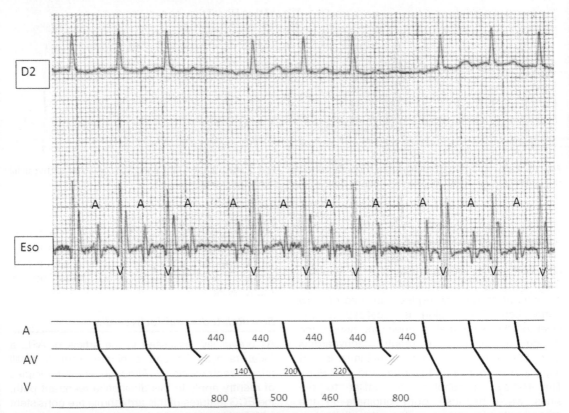

A			440	440	440	440	440			
AV				140	200	220				
V		800	500	460	800					

Fig. 17. Atrial Tachycardia miming atrial fibrillation. P wave isn't well evident in D2 and a variation of the RR cycle mimes atrial fibrillation; an esophageal (ESO) atrial lead shows atrial activity (A) in keeping with atrial tachycardia (A-A= 440 milliseconds) with second degree atrioventricular block (Wenckebach like sequence).

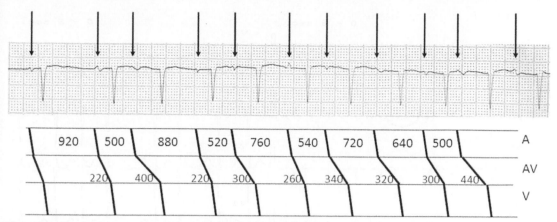

Fig. 18. Multifocal atrial tachycardias. Different P-wave (arrows) morphologies are evident.

of an isoelectric line cannot safely differentiate between flutters and micro-reentrant arrhythmias. These tachycardias are mostly related to the presence of scars and are often observed after AF ablation.

ATRIAL FIBRILLATION

The most common arrhythmia in clinical practice, atrial fibrillation, is characterized by a complete electrical atrial dyssynchrony (**Fig. 20**).

Atrial Activation in Atrial Fibrillation

ECG of AF is characterized by absence of an identifiable P wave, which is substituted with an incessant undulating electrical atrial activation, called the f wave; this has variable polarity and rate and complete absence of the isoelectric line. The voltage of the f wave can vary from a more recognizable wave, coarse AF to an almost flat line, fine AF (**Fig. 21**).

At times, periods of sporadic electrical organization are noted with discernable waves especially in

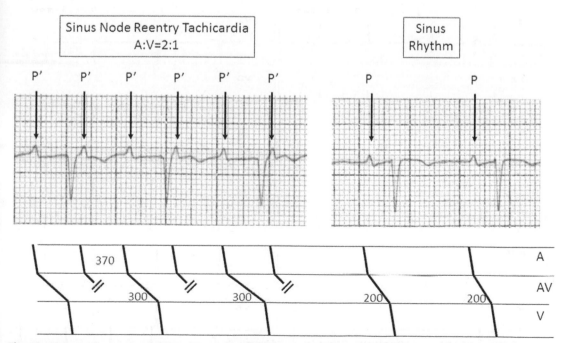

Fig. 19. Sinus node reentry tachycardia: a regular tachycardia (P′–P′ = 370 milliseconds) showing P′ wave similar to sinus P wave. During the tachycardia, 2:1 atrioventricular conduction is evident.

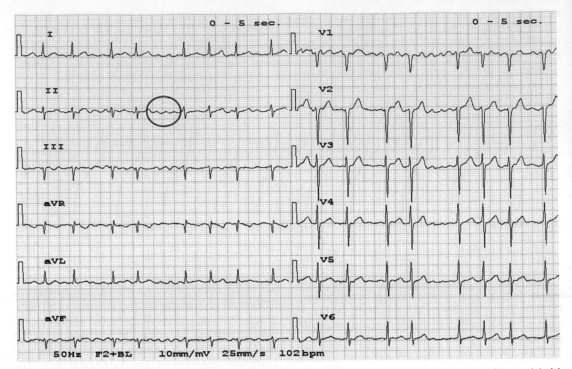

Fig. 20. Atrial fibrillation: the typical pattern of incessant undulating electrical atrial activation, f wave (*circle*), and complete absence of the isoelectric line. The RR interval is continuously variable.

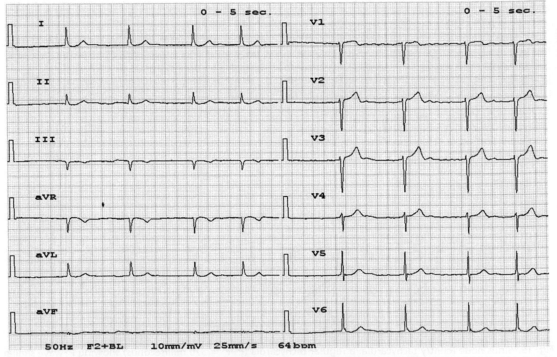

Fig. 21. Atrial fibrillation: low-amplitude fibrillation waves are present (fine atrial fibrillation).

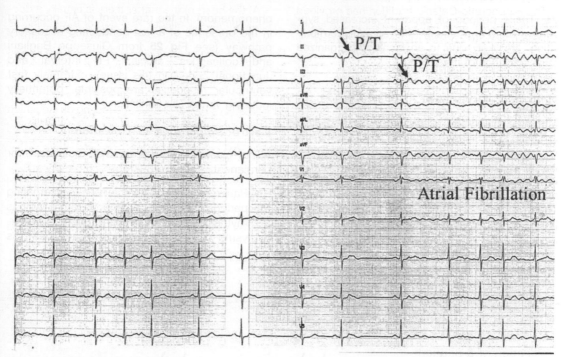

Fig. 22. Paroxysmal atrial fibrillation. Atrial fibrillation ends and starts again after ectopic beats (P/T phenomenon); see **Fig. 26** for further details.

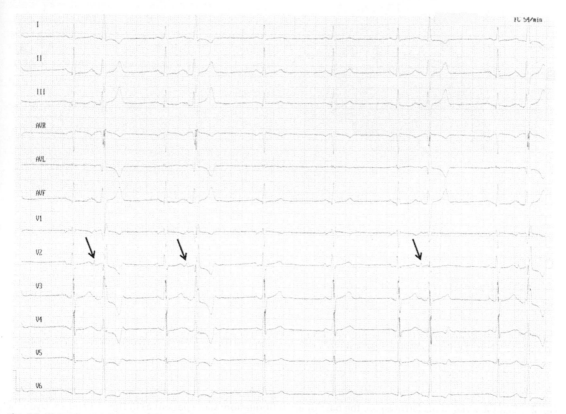

Fig. 23. Ectopic atrial beats (*arrows*) (conducted to the ventricles with bundle branch block) are the trigger for atrial fibrillation (**Figs. 24** and **25**).

V1. These periods of apparent increased synchrony, often erroneously referred as flutter/fibrillation, are likely due to an increased organized atrial activation of the CT.

Ventricular Response of Atrial Fibrillation

Marked R-R variation, often defined as irregularly irregular, is the other hallmark of AF. This unusual ventricular response is due to the concealed conduction of fibrillatory wavefronts, which, even if unable to propagate to the ventricles, modifies refractoriness of the AVN and its conduction. The overall QRS morphology is within normal limits, unless functional blocks due to short and long cycle variation supervenes (Ashman

phenomenon). In the rare event of AF occurring in the presence of a fast conducting accessory pathway (see **Fig 25** from Giuseppe Bagliani and colleagues' article, "PR Interval and Junctional Zone," in this issue), extremely fast ventricular responses are possible, potentially inducing ventricular fibrillation.

Electrocardiographic Classification

AF is classified as paroxysmal, persistent, or permanent.

- Paroxysmal AF is characterized by alternating periods of AF and spontaneous return to sinus rhythm (**Fig. 22**). A frequent trigger of paroxysms of AF is a premature atrial beat (as

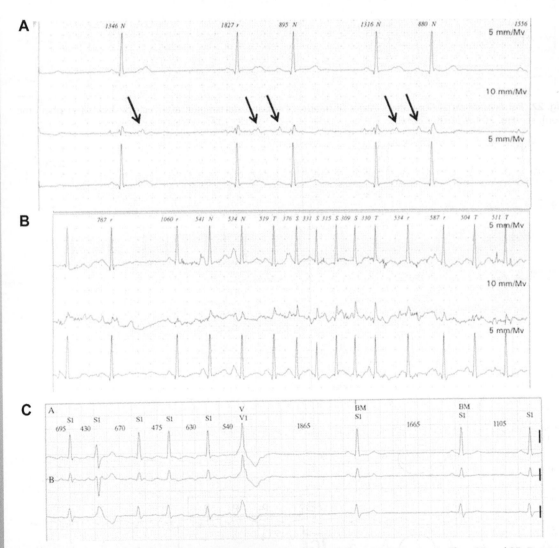

Fig. 24. Ectopic atrial beats (arrows) are the base of atrial fibrillation: same patient as in **Figs. 23** and **25**. Dynamic recording shows ectopic atrial beats not always conducted to the ventricles (*A*); paroxysmal atrial fibrillation stats (*B*) and ends (*C*).

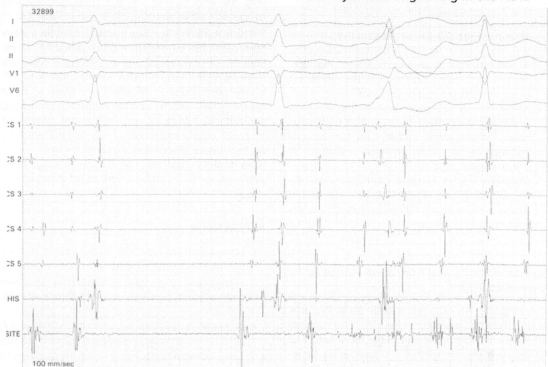

Fig. 25. Paroxysmal atrial fibrillation during electrophysiologic study.

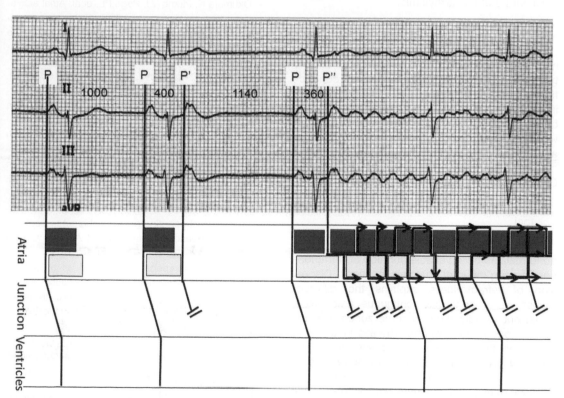

Fig. 26. Paroxysmal atrial fibrillation: atrial prematurity and dispersion of the atria refractoriness at base of paroxysmal atrial fibrillation. During sinus rhythm (P–P = 1000), an ectopic P′ beat is blocked at the level of AVN (P–P′ = 400 milliseconds). A long P′-P interval prolongs differently atrial refractoriness (*red and yellow tracts*); this dispersion of the refractoriness is the substrate for atrial fibrillation and the next ectopic beat (P″) can induce atypical AFL and then atrial fibrillation.

shown in **Figs. 23–25** recorded in the same individual), occurring with a critical relationship to the previous atrial depolarization (**Fig. 26**). This is particularly common in the presence of an abnormal sinus node function.

- AF is defined as persistent in the absence of spontaneous return to sinus rhythm. Restoration of the sinus rhythm can be accomplished with antiarrhythmic drugs or cardioversion.
- Permanent AF is the result of profound electrical and structural remodeling. The arrhythmia in this substrate cannot be converted to sinus rhythm

Mechanisms of Atrial Fibrillation Analyzed by 12-Lead ECG

Foci inducing AF originate mostly from the area around the atrial insertion of the PVs. The success of RFA eliminating AF is due to the focal nature of the trigger of this arrhythmia. Frequent and premature atrial contractions and runs of atrial tachycardia are other clinical manifestations of the focal nature of this arrhythmia.

- Atrial substrate: interatrial conduction delay

Conduction delays within the atria are instrumental in maintaining the multiple reentrant circuits typical of AF. Delays or blocks of interatrial conduction can be manifested via ECG with, respectively, increased duration of P wave, or 2 distinct P-wave components (bifid P) and a prolonged P duration with a terminal negative component (see **Figs. 5** and **6**; Giuseppe Bagliani and colleagues' article, "P Wave and the Substrates of Arrhythmias Originating in the Atria," in this issue).

- Dispersion of refractoriness and atrial ectopic foci

Atrial conduction delays can be due to structural abnormalities or to variable duration of refractoriness among different anatomic locations. Dispersion of refractoriness explains the different responses of anatomic contiguous areas to a wavefront of activation; in some zones, the impulse propagates normally, whereas in others it is blocked creating the basis for a reentrant circuit. The severity of dispersion of refractoriness is increased by variable stimulation frequency, as is the case during frequent atrial extrasystoles. Atrial premature contractions can, with this mechanism, modify the substrate refractoriness and trigger AF (see **Fig. 26**).

- Role of Autonomic Nervous System

The autonomic nervous system plays an important role in the triggering of paroxysmal AF. Modulations of both vagal and sympathetic tone are relevant in the induction of specific forms of AF: bradycardia-induced AF often observed at night from hypervagotonia and AF related to increased sympathetic drive during emotional stress or physical effort. Induction of AF is facilitated by an increased dispersion of refractoriness mediated by the heightened vagal tone and increased automaticity induced by augmented sympathetic drive.

REFERENCES

1. Ndrepepa G, Zrenner B, Deisenhofer I, et al. Relationship between surface electrocardiogram characteristics and endocardial activation sequence in patients with typical atrial flutter. Z Kardiol 2000;89: 527–37.
2. SippensGroenewegen A, Lesh MD, Roithinger FX, et al. Body surface mapping of counterclockwise and clockwise typical atrial flutter: a comparative analysis with endocardial activation sequence mapping. J Am Coll Cardiol 2000;35(5):1276–87.
3. Okumura K, Plumb VJ, Page PL, et al. Atrial activation sequence during atrial flutter in the canine pericarditis model and its effect on the polarity of the flutter wave in the electrocardiogram. J Am Coll Cardiol 1991;17:509–18.
4. Marine JE, Korley VJ, Obioha-Ngwu O, et al. Different patterns of interatrial conduction in clockwise and counterclockwise atrial flutter. Circulation 2001;104:1153–7.
5. Ashino S, Watanabe I, Okumura Y, et al. Change in atrial flutter wave morphology—insight into the sources of electrocardiographic variants in common atrial flutter. Pacing Clin Electrophysiol 2007;30: 1023–6.
6. Milliez P, Richardson AW, Obioha-Ngwu O, et al. Variable electrocardiographic characteristics of isthmus-dependent atrial flutter. J Am Coll Cardiol 2002;40:1125–32.
7. Zrenner B, Ndrepepa G, Karch M, et al. Schmitt block of the lower interatrial connections: insight into the sources of electrocardiographic diversities in common type atrial flutter. Pacing Clin Electrophysiol 2000;23:917–20.
8. Chugh A, Latchamsetty R, Oral H, et al. Characteristics of cavotricuspid isthmus–dependent atrial flutter after left atrial ablation of atrial fibrillation. Circulation 2006;113:609–15.
9. Sasaki K, Sasaki S, Kimura M, et al. Revisit of typical counterclockwise atrial flutter Wav in the ECG: electroanatomic studies on the determinant of the morphology. Pacing Clin Electrophysiol 2013;36: 978–87.

10. Yang Y, Cheng J, Bochoeyer A, et al. Atypical right atrial flutter patterns. Circulation 2001;103: 3092–8.

11. Yan SH, Cheng WJ, Wang LX, et al. Mechanisms of atypical flutter wave morphology in patients with isthmus-dependent atrial flutter. Heart Vessels 2009;24:211–8.

12. Tai CT, Huang JL, Lin YK, et al. Noncontact three-dimensional mapping and ablation of upper loop re-entry originating in the right atrium. J Am Coll Cardiol 2002;40(4):746–53.

13. Yuniadi Y, Tai CT, Lee KT, et al. A new electrocardiographic algorithm to differentiate upper loop re-entry from reverse typical atrial flutter. J Am Coll Cardiol 2005;46(3):524–8.

14. Ma W, Lu F, Wu D, et al. Cavotricuspid-dependent atrial flutter in Patients With prior atriotomy: 12-lead ECG interpretation and electroanatomical characteristics. J Cardiovasc Electrophysiol 2015;26:969–77.

15. Kistler PM, Kalman JM. Locating focal atrial tachycardias from P-wave morphology. Heart Rhythm 2005;2:561–4.

16. Gerstenfeld EP, Dixit S, Bala R, et al. Surface electrocardiogram characteristics of atrial tachycardias occurring after pulmonary vein isolation. Heart Rhythm 2007;4:1136–43.

PR Interval and Junctional Zone

Giuseppe Bagliani, MD[a,b,*], Domenico Giovanni Della Rocca, MD[c,d],
Luigi Di Biase, MD, PhD[d,e,f,g], Luigi Padeletti, MD[h,i]

KEYWORDS

- PR interval • Atrioventricular junction • Wenckebach periodicity • Accessory pathway
- Cardiac pre-excitation

KEY POINTS

- The atrioventricular junction is located within the triangle of Koch, an area in the low right atrium demarcated by the ostium of the coronary sinus, the tendon of Todaro, and the septal leaflet of the tricuspid valve.
- The sophisticated functions carried out by the atrioventricular junction are possible for the presence of a complex apparatus, made of specialized anatomic structures, cells with specific ion-channel expression, a well-organized spatial distribution of connexins, cells with intrinsic automatism, and a rich autonomic innervation.
- The PR interval represents the time from onset of atrial depolarization to onset of ventricular depolarization, encompassing the entire atrioventricular conduction system.
- Cardiac pre-excitation is present when the ventricles are activated via an accessory pathway, anticipating the normal sequence of electrical activation of the heart.

INTRODUCTION

This article focuses our attention on the atrioventricular (AV) junction, which is a pivotal component of the cardiac conduction system, a key electrical relay site between the atria and the ventricles. The AV junction does not simply act as a passive conduction system linking the atria to the ventricles, but is a sophisticated regulatory system, which determines when to promote, delay, or block the conduction of atrial depolarizations to the ventricles. In healthy patients, the AV junction optimizes the AV delay. During normal sinus rhythm, atrial contraction actively contributes to the ventricular end-diastolic filling; as such, the AV delay changes based on the heart rate, with an inverse relationship between AV interval and sinus rate. Additionally, cells in the AV junction may serve as an escape pacemaker; this may occur during periods of sinus node pauses. Rarely, a junctional rhythm can take over, usually during acute illnesses, sympathetic overdrive, or after cardiac surgery.

THE PR INTERVAL

The PR interval represents the time from onset of atrial depolarization to onset of ventricular depolarization, encompassing the entire AV conduction

No relevant conflicts to disclose.
[a] Arrhythmology Unit, Cardiology Department, Foligno General Hospital, Via Massimo Arcamone, 06034 Foligno (PG), Italy; [b] Cardiovascular Diseases Department, University of Perugia, Piazza Menghini 1, 06129 Perugia Italy; [c] Department of Cardiovascular Medicine, University of Rome Tor Vergata, Rome, Italy; [d] Texas Cardiac Arrhythmia Institute, St. David's Medical Center, 3000 N IH 35, Ste 700, Austin, TX 78705, USA; [e] Department of Biomedical Engineering, University of Texas, Austin, TX, USA; [f] Montefiore Medical Center, Albert Einstein College of Medicine, Bronx, NY, USA; [g] Department of Clinical and Experimental Medicine, University of Foggia, Foggia, Italy; [h] Heart and Vessels Department, University of Florence, Largo Brambilla, 3, 50134 Florence, Italy; [i] IRCCS Multimedica, Cardiology Department, Via Milanese, 300, 20099 Sesto San Giovanni, Italy
* Corresponding author. Arrhythmology Clinic Unit, Cardiology Department, Foligno General Hospital, Foligno, Italy.
E-mail address: giuseppe.bagliani@tim.it

Card Electrophysiol Clin 9 (2017) 411–433
http://dx.doi.org/10.1016/j.ccep.2017.05.003
1877-9182/17/© 2017 Elsevier Inc. All rights reserved.

system (**Fig. 1**). There are 3 distinct conductive elements:

- *Internodal tracts:* The sinus impulse travels from the sinus node to the AV node via preferential activation of 3 specialized conduction pathways, the so-called anterior, middle, and posterior internodal tracts. These are located in the right atrium, and, as such, the impulse reaches the AV node before all atrial myocytes have depolarized, that is, the AV node is activated before the end of the P wave.
- *AV junction:* The impulse then travels through the AV junction, which encompasses the AV node and the His bundle, before it branches.
- *His bundle branches and Purkinje fibers:* Finally, the impulse begins to activate the ventricular specialized conduction system, namely the 2 bundle branches (right and left) and their ramifications (the Purkinje network). From a strictly anatomo-electrophysiologic point of view, this segment is part of the ventricles, but because its electrical activity cannot be recorded, its activation falls in the PR interval.

On the surface electrocardiogram (ECG), the PR interval is measured from the beginning of the P wave to the beginning of the QRS complex. To avoid interpretation errors and to ensure the reproducibility of the PR interval measurements, it is important to identify the earliest onset of the P wave and the earliest onset of the QRS complex. Frequently, these 2 temporal points are not in the same derivation; therefore, the PR interval should be calculated using a 12-lead ECG. Measurements performed on a single lead can be misleading if there is loss of electrical amplitude of the P wave or the QRS complex. For example, the P wave can be isoelectric in those leads in which the atrial activation wavefront is perpendicular, leading to underestimation of the PR interval (**Fig. 2**).

ANATOMY OF THE ATRIOVENTRICULAR JUNCTION

The sophisticated functions carried out by the AV junction are possible for the presence of a complex apparatus, made of specialized anatomic

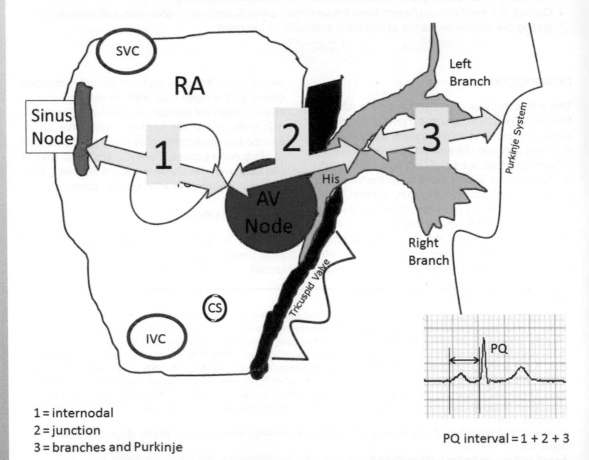

1 = internodal
2 = junction
3 = branches and Purkinje

PQ interval = 1 + 2 + 3

Fig. 1. AV conduction system. CS, coronary sinus; IVC, inferior vena cava; RA, right atrium; SVC, superior vena cava.

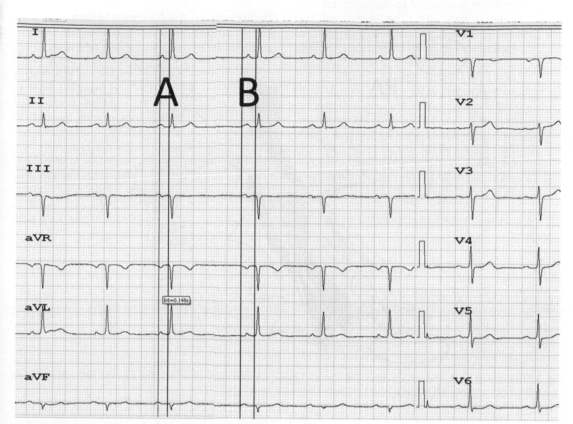

Fig. 2. How to measure the PR interval (see text for description).

structures, cells with specific ion-channel expression, a well-organized spatial distribution of intercellular junctions (connexins), cells with intrinsic automatism, and a rich autonomic innervation.[1–3]

The AV junction is located within the triangle of Koch (**Fig. 3**), an area in the low right atrium, demarcated by the ostium of the coronary sinus, the tendon of Todaro, and the septal leaflet of the tricuspid valve.[1–3] Structurally, the AV junction comprises 3 portions: the atrial inputs to the AV node, the compact AV node, and the bundle of His.

Atrial cells do not communicate directly with the compact AV node but only through specific atrionodal connections that can be found in the triangle of Koch.[4,5] More specifically, these inputs comprise 2 functionally distinct cell populations (see **Fig. 3**):

- Transitional cells, located in the superior and middle part of the triangle of Koch, extending toward the fossa ovalis
- Cells of the inferior nodal extensions (INE), located in the middle and inferior part of the triangle of Koch, extending toward the coronary sinus ostium, parallel to the septal leaflet of the tricuspid valve

Although histologically these cells are similar (relatively small and surrounded connective tissue), there are important molecular and electrophysiological differences. More specifically, different connexins (Cx) are expressed by the 2 cell populations. There are 4 Cx isoforms in the human heart, with different conductive properties[6–8]: Cx40 (highly conductive), Cx43 (average), Cx45 (low), and Cx31.9 (ultralow—poorly expressed). The atrial myocardium expresses high levels of Cx40 and Cx43, the transitional cells express intermediate levels of Cx40 and Cx43, whereas the cells of the INE express low levels of Cx40 and Cx43 and high levels of Cx45. This differential expression might explain some of the features of the AV junction and the existence of a functional compartmentalization, which parallels the structural one. Additionally, gene expression studies have found that compact AV node and INE cells express high levels of $Ca_v1.3$, responsible for the L-type calcium current, whereas transitional and His bundle cells express higher levels of protein $Na_v1.5$, responsible for the fast upstroke sodium current.[9–12] Interestingly, INE cells also show high levels of HCN4,[12] which is responsible for the hyperpolarization-activated "funny" (I_f) current

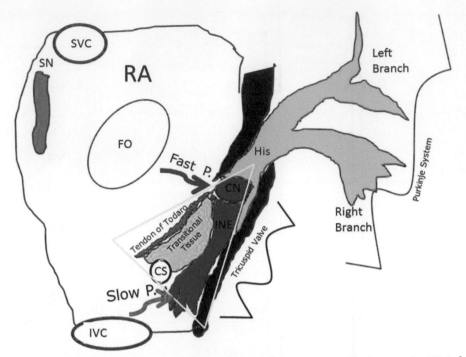

Fig. 3. Triangle of Koch and AV junction. CN, compact node; CS, coronary sinus; FO, fossa ovalis; IVC, inferior vena cava; RA, right atrium; SN, sinus node; SVC, superior vena cava.

and might explain how the cells in the AV junction are capable of spontaneous depolarization, acting as an independent pacemaker and as a site of enhanced automaticity.[10]

The compact AV node is located at the apex of the triangle of Koch and is the site at which conduction delay is the greatest. Cells in the compact AV node are compact and spindle shaped and on a molecular level are similar to the INE cells: they express high levels of Cx45 and Ca$_v$1.3, and low levels of Cx40 and Cx43, explaining the slow conduction properties.[9,11,12]

The bundle of His is the lowest and fastest component of the AV junction. After passing the AV node, the impulse travels fast through the His bundle, its branches, and the Purkinje network, activating both ventricles almost simultaneously. The high speed of the His bundle[9,13] can be explained by the presence of a high concentration of connexins with high conductivity (Cx40 and Cx43). An interesting observation is that there are 2 functionally distinct segments of the His bundle, superior and inferior,[13] that are selectively activated by the depolarization wavefront coming from either the transitional zone or the INE,[14,15] respectively (**Fig. 4**). This phenomenon can be seen by recording the upper and lower part of the His bundle: when the atrial impulse travels though the transitional zone (superior input), the

superior part of the His bundle is activated first and voltage is higher in the upper electrodes, whereas when the INE is used, the inferior His bundle is activated before its superior portion, and the highest voltage is recorded in the lower electrodes.[16] For this reason, this phenomenon is also called *His alternans*.[15,17]

ELECTROPHYSIOLOGY OF THE ATRIOVENTRICULAR JUNCTION
PR Variation, the Result of Preferential and Concealed Conduction

The analysis of PR interval can provide specific information about the AV junction complex activation. During sinus tachycardia, the normal delay of conduction through the AV node is reduced. Sympathetic activation increases the AV nodal conduction velocity, reducing the time between atrial and ventricular activation.[18,19] As a result, the PR interval is shorter, maximizing the end-diastolic ventricular filling via a well-timed atrial contraction (atrial kick). On the other hand, when the atrial rate is too high, such as in the case of atrial arrhythmias, the AV junction functions as a gatekeeper, limiting the impulses that reach the ventricle by prolonging the PR interval up to AV block. These phenomena are the result of a complex interaction between the complex structures

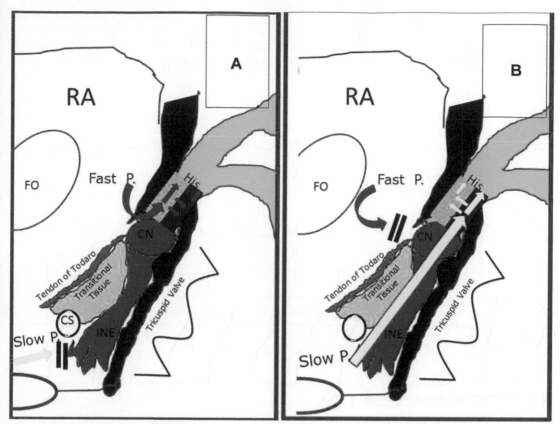

Fig. 4. His bundle activation with atrial pulse coming from the fast pathway (*A*). His bundle activation with atrial pulse coming from the slow pathway (*B*) (see text for description). CN, compact node; CS, coronary sinus; FO, fossa ovalis; RA, right atrium.

that comprise the AV junction and autonomic innervation. More specifically, the superior input, composed of transitional cells, depolarizes fast via the Na-current, a high depolarizing flow, which takes longer to repolarize; instead, the inferior input is composed of cells that depolarize via the slow Ca-current, with a shorter repolarization time. Autonomic innervation influences the conduction through the AV junction conduction by modulating the refractory period. During normal sinus rhythm, the atrial impulse activates preferentially the superior transitional zone, whereas activation of the INE is concealed: the PR is normal. During sinus tachycardia, the enhanced sympathetic tone facilitates conduction through the superior input, explaining shortening of the PR interval. In case of a premature atrial contraction (PAC) or atrial tachycardia, without corresponding enhanced sympathetic activation, the atrial activation wavefront reaches the superior input while it is still refractory (**Fig. 5**). The impulse then travels through the INE with a suddenly longer PR interval. Moreover, there is progressive prolongation of the PR interval as the prematurity of the

PAC increases (**Fig. 6**). This can be explained by the presence of a conductive continuum through the different atrio-nodal inputs, with gradually slowing conduction times. This is not surprising; although morphologically distinct, the transitional zone and INE are not completely isolated and interact owing to anatomic proximity and cellular overlapping. Finally, if the impulse is too premature, it reaches the INE when it's still refractory, and it cannot be conducted down the compact AV node up to the ventricles; the PAC is blocked.

Continuous Conduction: Progressive PR Prolongation and Wenckebach Periodicity as a Paraphysiologic Phenomenon

This selective concealed conduction to different atrio-nodal inputs can explain other commonly observed phenomena.[20–22] During dynamic ECG recordings, for a set atrial rate, it is not uncommon to observe a progressive prolongation of the PR interval until an atrial impulse is not propagated (second degree, type I AV block, or Luciani-Wenckebach phenomenon). Characteristically,

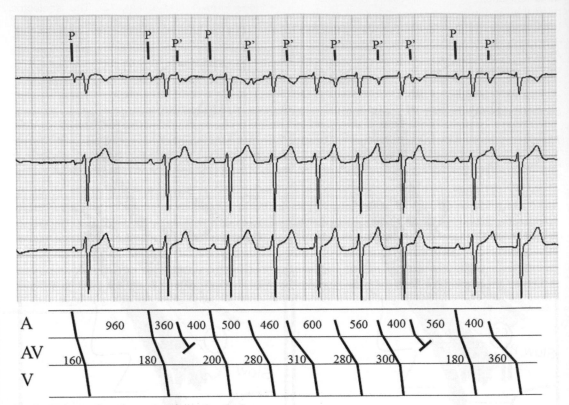

Fig. 5. PR interval prolongation following PACs.

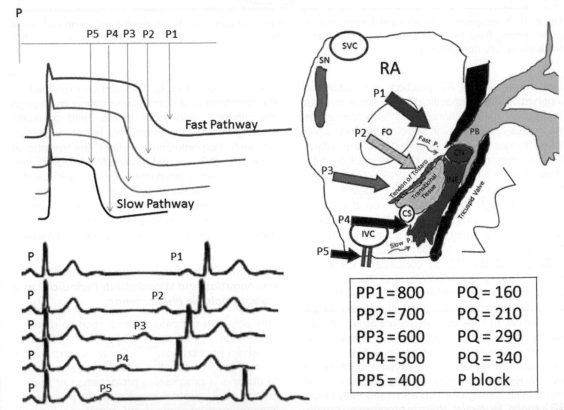

Fig. 6. Progressive prolongation of the PR interval as prematurity of the PAC increases. CN, compact node; CS, coronary sinus; IVC, inferior vena cava; RA, right atrium; SN, sinus node; SVC, superior vena cava

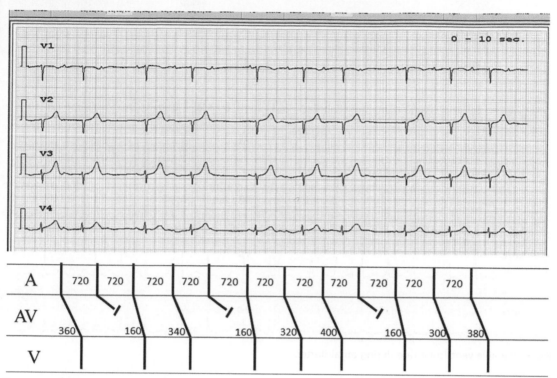

Fig. 7. Luciani-Wenckebach periodicity.

the PR interval is shorter in the first beat after the nonconducted impulse (**Fig. 7**). This can be explained by a progressive conductive shift from the superior to the inferior atrio-nodal input, a sequence that is restored after the blocked beat, when conduction resumes over the superior fast-conducting pathway (normal PR). Additionally, a selective concealed conduction can explain the variation in the ventricular rate observed during atrial fibrillation (**Fig. 8**) and atrial flutter (**Fig. 9**).

Discontinuous Conduction: Dual Pathway and the Substrate of Nodal Re-entry

AV conduction is usually continuous, that is, with progressive prolongation of the PR interval with higher degrees of prematurity. However, it is not infrequent to observe a significant prolongation of the PR interval with minimal or any variation of the atrial cycle length. This finding indicates the presence of 2 electrophysiologically distinct

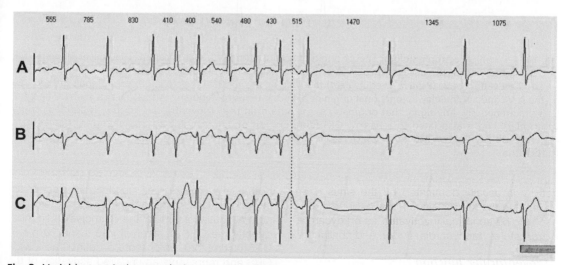

Fig. 8. Variable ventricular rate during atrial fibrillation.

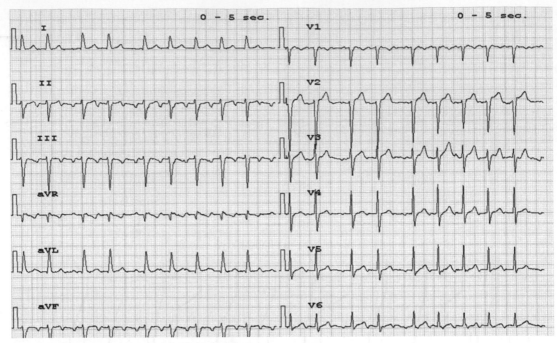

Fig. 9. Variable ventricular rate during atrial flutter.

conduction pathways, the so-called fast and slow pathway (**Fig. 10**). Anatomically, the slow pathway is hypothesized to be part of the INE, expressing an alternative L-type calcium channel isoform, responsible for slower Ca^{2+}-dependent conduction times. The fast pathway is thought to be composed of transitional cells that extend superiorly and posteriorly to the compact AV node, with a relative higher expression of Cx40, Cx43, and $Na_v1.5$, explaining the faster conduction properties.[9,11,12] However, experimental data are still conflicting. Another possible explanation of the shorter conduction delay is circuit length, which is shorter compared with that of the slow pathway.[23–25] Irrespective of the explanation, the presence of a dual AV node physiology can be easily proved in the electrophysiology laboratory with programmed stimulation when a prolongation of the PR interval of at least 50 milliseconds after a 10-millisecond decrement of the premature atrial stimulation. Of note, this jump is preceded by progressive prolongation of the PR interval, which

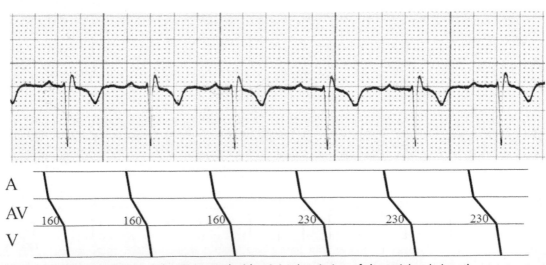

Fig. 10. Significant variation of the PR interval with minimal variation of the atrial cycle length.

means that its origin is in a structure outside to the normal atrio-nodal inputs. More specifically, it is the expression of a very slow conducing pathway, different from the INE. In rare cases, conduction through this pathway is so slow that the same atrial impulse can be conducted twice to the ventricles (**Fig. 11**). The presence of a dual AV node physiology means only that the subject has the potential substrate for re-entry. The clinical tachycardia (AV nodal re-entrant tachycardia) can develop only if the premature impulse can travel back the fast pathway and down again the slow pathway perpetuating the re-entry mechanism.

Retrograde Conduction in the Atrioventricular Junction

During retrograde conduction, the impulse propagates from the ventricles to the atria through the AV junction. Retrograde conduction is uncommon,[26] with block occurring at distal sites (compact AV node or lower). When present, retrograde conduction occurs preferentially over the fast transitional cells (**Fig. 12**). Well-timed ventricular beats can also highlight a concealed retrograde conduction over the transitional cells,[26] as evidenced by PR prolongation in the first sinus beat that follows the ventricular beat (**Fig. 13**).

The phenomenon is most evident during atrial fibrillation, in which ventricular ectopic beats are often followed by a significant prolongation of the RR interval (**Fig. 14**).

CARDIAC PRE-EXCITATION

Normally, the AV junction is the only connection between the atria and the ventricles. However, in some individuals, there are additional muscle bundles located around the AV grove, through which the electrical impulse can bypass the AV junction (the so-called accessory pathways [AP] or bypass tracts). Cardiac pre-excitation is present when the ventricles are activated via an accessory pathway, anticipating the normal sequence of electrical activation of the heart.

The most common form of cardiac pre-excitation is secondary to the presence of fast-conducting AP that directly connect the atrial and ventricular myocardium (Kent bundles). When this AP conducts anterogradely (manifest pre-excitation), the ventricles are activated by 2 wavefronts, propagating from the normal and the accessory pathways (**Fig. 15**). Given the faster conduction, the ventricles are first activated by the AP resulting in the delta wave formation, then the normal conduction through the His-

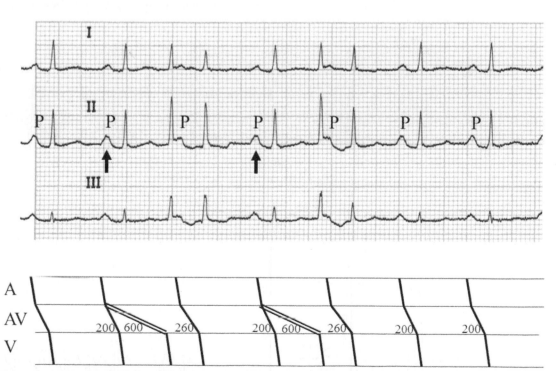

Fig. 11. A 1:2 Atrio-Ventricular conduction in a patient with dual AV node physiology. Occasionally the same P wave (*arrow*) is conducted twice to the ventricles.

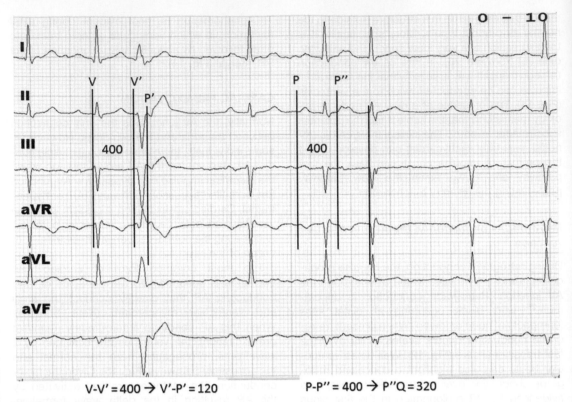

$$V\text{-}V' = 400 \rightarrow V'\text{-}P' = 120 \qquad P\text{-}P'' = 400 \rightarrow P''Q = 320$$

Fig. 12. Retrograde P waves.

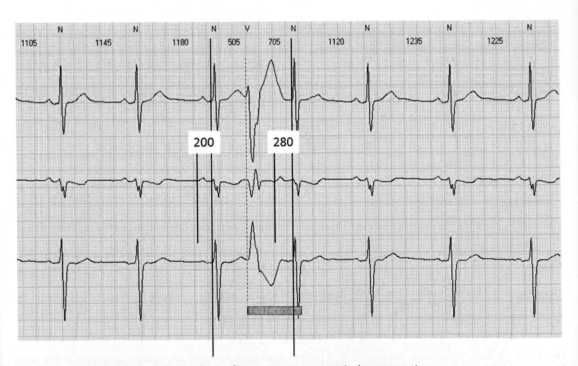

Fig. 13. PR prolongation in the sinus beat after a premature ventricular contraction.

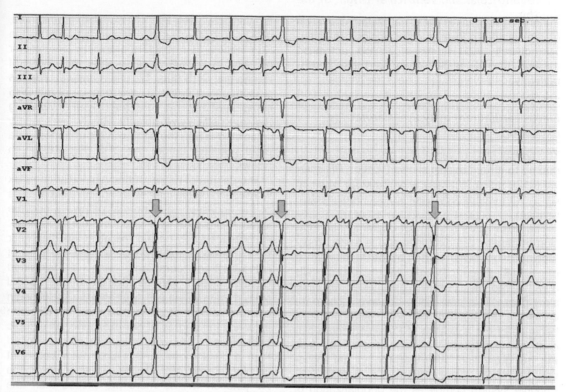

Fig. 14. Premature ventricular contractions (*arrows*) during atrial fibrillation followed by significant prolongation of the RR interval.

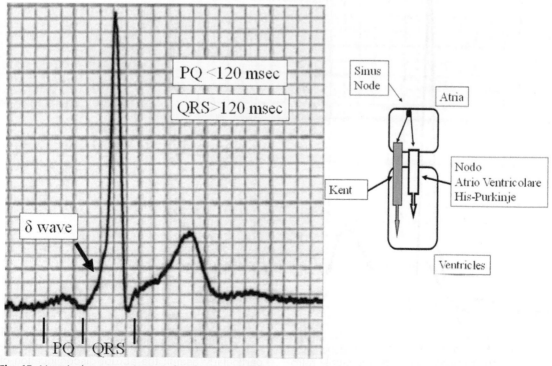

Fig. 15. Ventricular pre-excitation during sinus rhythm.

Purkinje system takes over, completing activation of the ventricles in a more physiologic manner. The overall result is fusion of the activation through the AP (delta wave), and the normal pathway.

Electrocardiogram of Typical Cardiac Pre-excitation

The typical ECG of ventricular pre-excitation secondary to a Kent bundle shows (1) short PR interval (<120 msec), (2) delta wave, and (3) widened QRS with secondary ventricular repolarization changes.

The delta wave is the most characteristic ECG sign of cardiac pre-excitation and is a low amplitude and slope signal caused by the depolarization of a small amount of ventricular myocardial cells (**Fig. 16**, red line). In some cases, after this initial slow phase, it is possible to observe a sharp increase in the slope of the delta wave probably because of the activation of Purkinje fibers adjacent to ventricular insertion of the AP (see **Fig. 16**, green line). After that, the normal activation wavefront coming from the normal His-Purkinje system completes the depolarization of

the ventricles (see **Fig. 16**, blue line). Sometimes, activation of the Purkinje system adjacent to the Kent bundle can generate a unidirectional vector resulting in R or S waves greater than those of the normal QRS (**Fig. 17**, green arrows). For this reason, only the first 40 milliseconds of the QRS complex should be considered when evaluating the true delta wave polarity. Rarely, and usually in isolated leads, the delta wave can appear as a rapid potential before the QRS (**Fig. 18**, green arrow).

The degree of fusion of the ventricular complex will depend on the intrinsic conductive capabilities of the accessory and normal pathways and the location of the AP with respect to the sinus node. A right-sided AP, having the atrial insertion near the sinus node, will produce a greater degree of pre-excitation compared with a left-sided pathway, which can be invisible during normal sinus rhythm (latent AP). Similarly, the site of origin and prematurity of an ectopic atrial impulse can influence the degree of pre-excitation. An ectopic beat closer to the AP will be more pre-excited than a distant one, and a premature beat that is blocked or has slow conduction over the AV junction will be more pre-excited than one

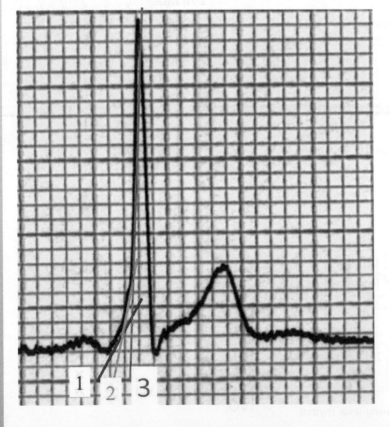

Fig. 16. Delta wave (see text for description).

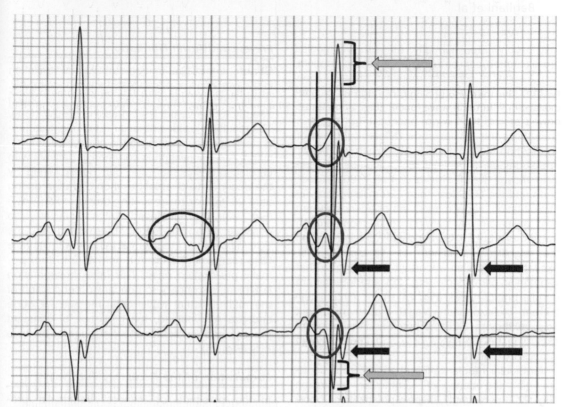

Fig. 17. Alternant Ventricular Preexcitation: a normal PR / normal QRS (*blue circle*) is followed by a short PR / wide QRS (*red circle*). The activation of the Purkinje system adjacent to the Kent bundle generates a taller R wave (superior *green arrow*) and a deeper S waves (*inferior green arrow*). The blue arrows indicate the late activation of the ventricles by the His-Purkinje system.

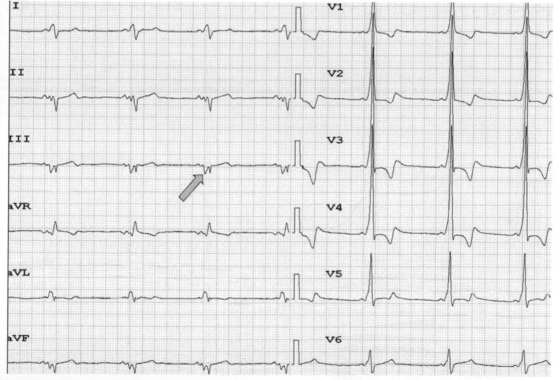

Fig. 18. Fixed Ventricular pre-excitation (*arrow*).

that is conducted normally. As such, ventricular pre-excitation can be dynamic; the same patient can display a constant manifest pre-excitation pattern (see **Fig. 18**) or different degrees of pre-excitation (intermittent pre-excitation). Sometimes only a single beat is pre-excited (**Fig. 19**), and sometimes the AP can show different degrees of conduction block (see **Fig. 17**). When ventricular pre-excitation is minimal, ECG findings may be insignificant; the PR interval can be ≥120 milliseconds and the QRS less than 120 milliseconds. In this situation, vagal maneuvers or adenosine can help by selectively slowing conduction through the AV node but not the bundle of Kent, unmasking the significant findings of ventricular pre-excitation. It is also important to recognize that ventricular parasystole (**Fig. 20**) and intermittent bundle branch block (**Fig. 21**) might mimic intermittent pre-excitation. Vagal maneuvers might help, as they result in AV block and dissociation, excluding the presence of a sodium-dependent accessory pathway.

Ventricular repolarization changes are secondary to alterations of ventricular activation (**Fig. 22**). Interestingly, these repolarization abnormalities may persist even after normal AV junction activation is restored (for example, in case of intermittent ventricular pre-excitation or after ablation). This is the so-called cardiac electrical memory, which might last for days, leading to an erroneous diagnosis of ischemia or ventricular overload.

Pre-excited Atrial Fibrillation

Of note, the ECG is unique during atrial fibrillation in the presence of a manifest, fast-conducting AP. In this scenario, the AP allows for rapid conduction directly to the ventricles bypassing the AV node. The resulting rapid ventricular rates might degenerate in ventricular tachycardia or ventricular fibrillation. Atrial fibrillation is common in patients with cardiac pre-excitation and can be explained by the occurrence of atrial desynchronization during atrio ventricular reciprocating tachycardia (AVRT) (**Fig. 23**), but enhanced automaticity is also possible (**Fig. 24**). During pre-excited AF, the ECG displays an irregular RR interval with variable QRS morphologies, from a normal QRS to maximally pre-excited ones. This latter phenomenon is typical, secondary to concealed conduction of the multiple atrial wavefronts into the AV node and the AP. Instead, the presence of constant pre-excitation indicates the presence of multiple APs (**Fig. 25**).

Localization of the Accessory Pathway

In the presence of manifest ventricular pre-excitation, it is possible to estimate the location of the AP by analyzing the delta wave polarity in the first 40 milliseconds of the pre-excited QRS, when ventricular conduction occurs exclusively through the AP.[27] To help visualize the correlation between the anatomic site of an AP and its ECG

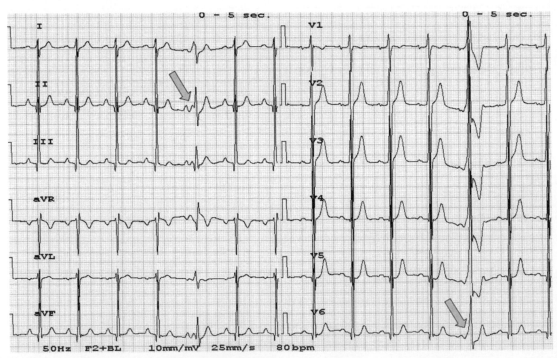

Fig. 19. Intermittent ventricular pre-excitation (*arrow*).

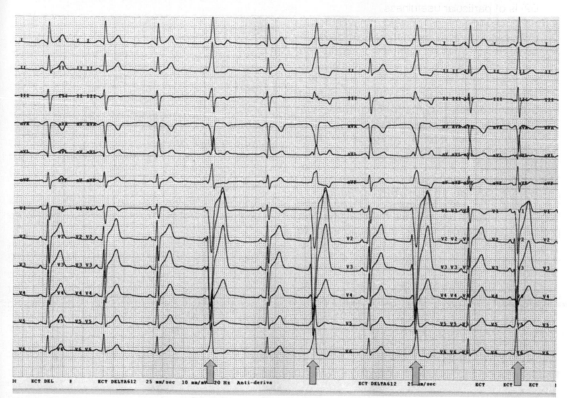

Fig. 20. Ventricular parasystole (*arrow*) mimicking intermittent ventricular pre-excitation.

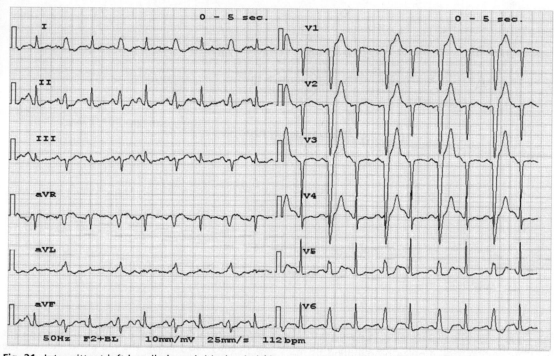

Fig. 21. Intermittent left bundle branch block mimicking intermittent ventricular pre-excitation.

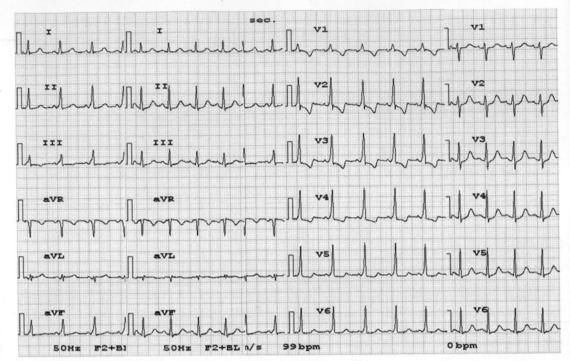

Fig. 22. Repolarization changes secondary to ventricular pre-excitation.

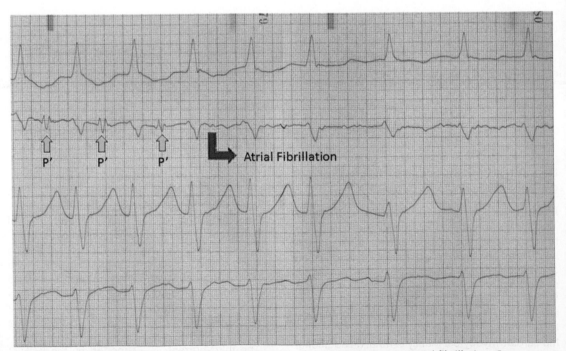

Fig. 23. Spontaneous degeneration of Atrio Ventricular Re-entry Tachycardia into atrial fibrillation. Green arrows indicate the activation of the atria during atrio-ventricular re-entry tachycardia. The red arrow indicate the degeneration in atrial fibrillation.

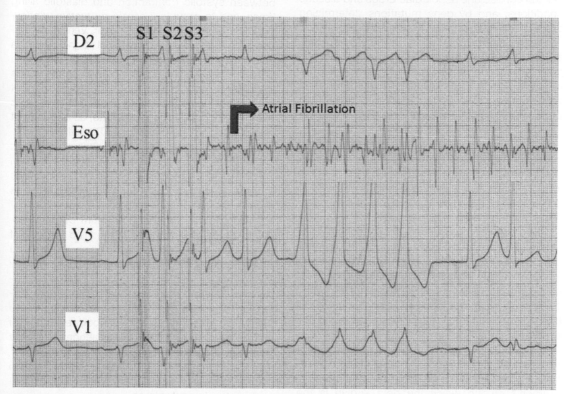

Fig. 24. Induction of pre-excited atrial fibrillation by atrial pacing. During sinus rhythm, three atrial stimuli are delivered at esophageal left atrial level. Esophageal lead (Eso) shows atrial fibrillation (*red arrow*) with the typical pattern of activation. The QRS complexes shows inconstant ventricular pre-excitation.

pattern, we should remember that the left ventricle is positioned higher and posteriorly, whereas the right ventricle faces downward and forward.

Roughly, a positive delta wave in V1 (a right precordial lead) is typical of a left-sided AP, whereas a negative delta wave is typical of right-sided AP (**Fig. 26**).

A left lateral AP activates the ventricles with a vector directed from left to right, top to bottom, and posterior to anterior. The delta wave is therefore negative in I and aVL; positive in the II, III, and aVF; and positive in V1 (**Fig. 27**). The left precordial leads can display a negative or positive delta wave, but the R-wave amplitude decreases from V4 to V6, as the AP activation vector is directed to the right.

A right lateral AP generates an activation vector directed from right to left, bottom to top, and anterior to posterior. The delta wave is positive in I and aVL, negative in III, negative in V1, and positive in V6 (**Fig. 28**).

An antero-septal AP generates a vector directed downward, to the left, and posteriorly. The delta wave is therefore positive in I, II, and III and negative in V1 to V3, where the ventricular complexes are exclusively negative (QS) (**Fig. 29**). A delta wave positive only in V1 and V2 indicates a para-Hisian AP.

Postero-septal APs are characterized by a vector of ventricular activation directed from the bottom to the top and to the left (**Figs. 30** and **31**). The delta wave is negative in the inferior leads, positive in I and aVL, and positive in the left precordial leads. To differentiate between right and left postero-septal pathway, the polarity of the delta wave in V1 is key; it will be negative in a right-sided pathway (see **Fig. 30**) and positive in a left-sided one (see **Fig. 31**) and will give a positive delta wave in the same lead V1. Multiple APs can be suspected when there are 2 distinct morphologies of ventricular pre-excitation during sinus rhythm or pre-excited atrial fibrillation (see **Fig. 25**).

Rare Variants of Cardiac Pre-excitation

Atypical APs are those pathways that bypass the AV junction but are not nonrapidly conducting or connecting the atrial and ventricular myocardium near the AV groove. When evident on the ECG, they might result in characteristic patterns of ventricular pre-excitation: the Mahaim type, with a normal PR and a pre-excited QRS (usually with

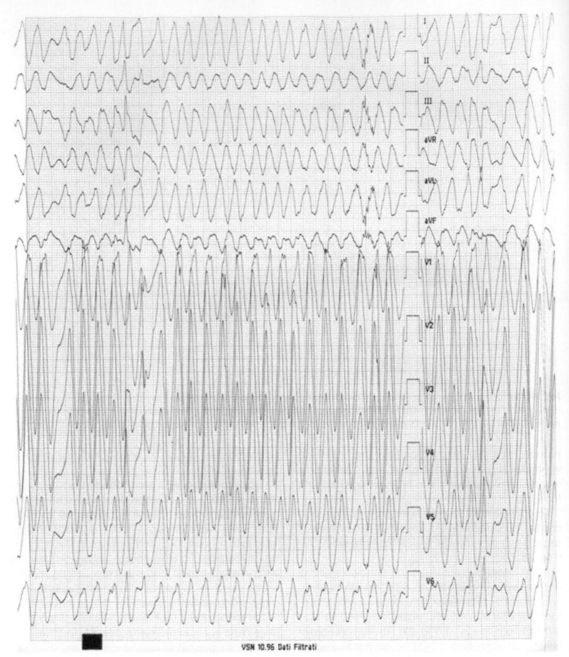

VSN 10.96 Dati Filtrati

Fig. 25. Pre-excited atrial fibrillation. The presence of a constant and maximal ventricular pre-excitation is indicative of multiple APs.

left bundle branch block morphology; **Fig. 32**) and the James type, with short PR and a normal QRS complex (**Fig. 33**). Mahaim fibers connect the atrium to the His (atrio-Hisian) or the fascicles (atrio-fascicular), the node to the fascicles (nodo-fascicular) or the ventricle (nodo-ventricular), or the fascicles to the ventricles (fasciculoventricular). The most common type of Mahaim pre-excitation is that involving a long, decrementally conducting APs located in the lateral or anterior tricuspid annulus, connecting the right atrium to the right bundle, close to the moderator band. This atrio-fascicular AP is essentially a second AV conduction system, that, when recorded during an electrophysiology study, displays a small, sharp potential similar to that of the bundle of His. James fibers are atrio-nodal APs that connect the atrium to the compact AV node. Their

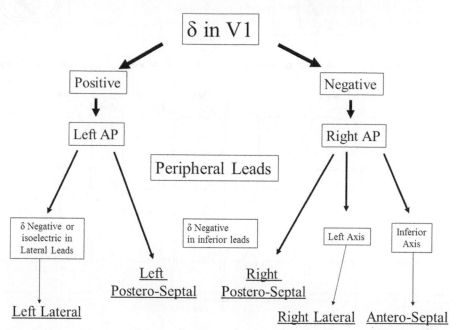

Fig. 26. Stepwise algorithm to determine the location of accessory pathways on a 12-lead ECG with ventricular pre-excitation.

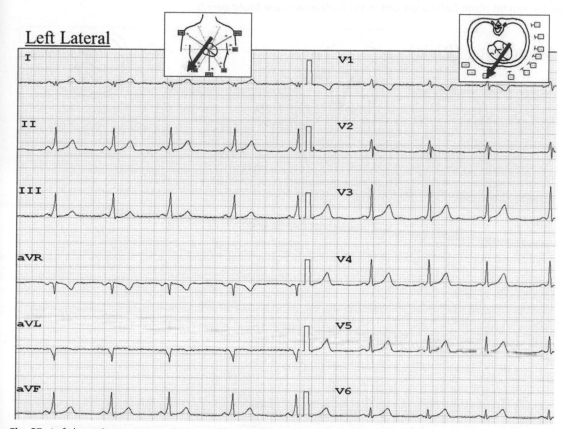

Fig. 27. Left lateral accessory pathway. The red arrow indicate the vector direction of ventricular pre-excitation on the frontal plane (*left panel*) and in the horizontal plane (*right panel*).

Right Lateral

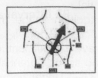
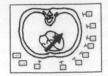

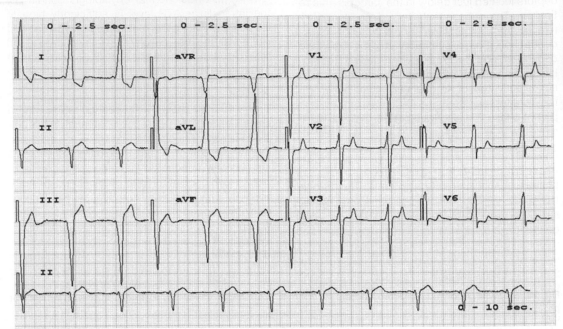

Fig. 28. Right lateral accessory pathway. The red arrow indicate the vector direction of ventricular pre-excitation on the frontal plane (*left panel*) and in the horizontal plane (*right panel*).

Anteroseptal (Right)

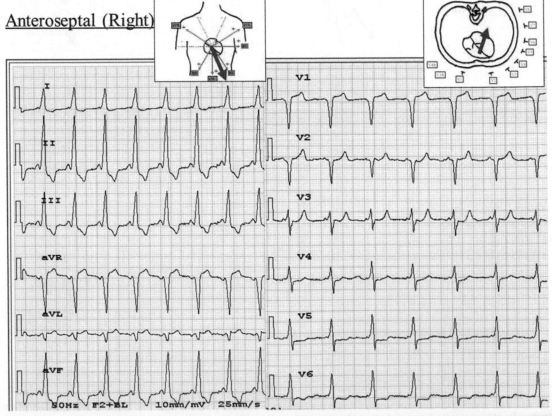

Fig. 29. Antero-septal accessory pathway. The red arrow indicate the vector direction of ventricular pre-excitation on the frontal plane (*left panel*) and in the horizontal plane (*right panel*).

Right Postero-Septal

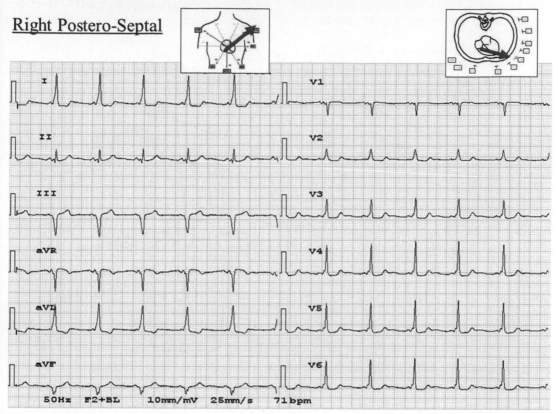

Fig. 30. Right postero-septal accessory pathway. The red arrow indicate the vector direction of ventricular pre-excitation on the frontal plane (*left panel*) and in the horizontal plane (*right panel*).

Left Postero-Septal

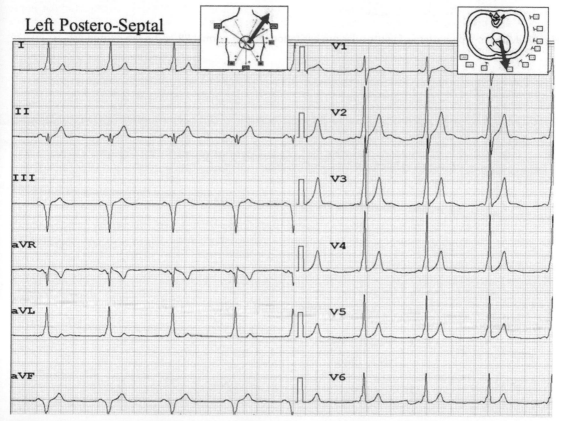

Fig. 31. Left postero-septal accessory pathway. The red arrow indicate the vector direction of ventricular pre-excitation on the frontal plane (*left panel*) and in the horizontal plane (*right panel*).

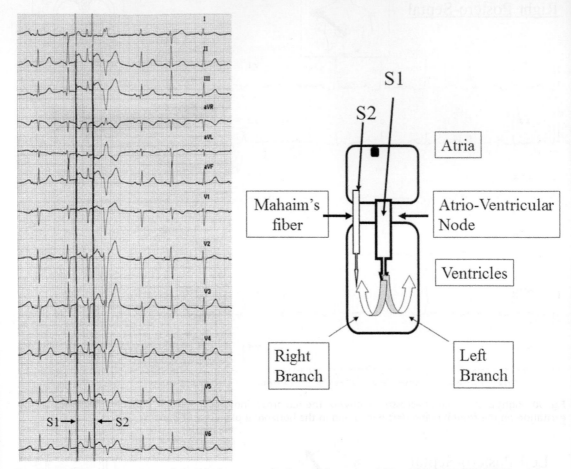

Fig. 32. Mahaim-type pattern of ventricular pre-excitation, with a normal PR and a pre-excited QRS.

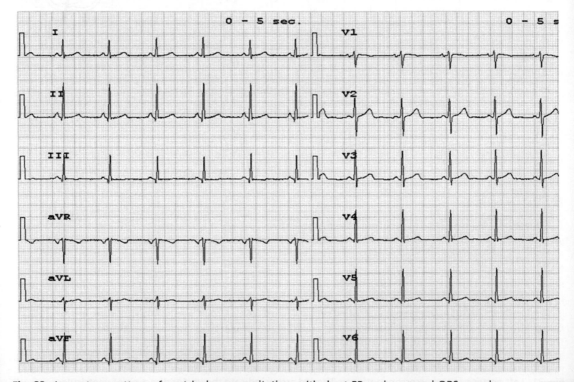

Fig. 33. James-type pattern of ventricular pre-excitation, with short PR and a normal QRS complex.

existence is debated, as a short PR interval and a normal QRS can be simply explained by a heightened sympathetic tone or an AV node with limited filtering capabilities (so-called immature AV node).

REFERENCES

1. Chang BC, Schuessler RB, Stone CM, et al. Computerized activation sequence mapping of the human atrial septum. Ann Thorac Surg 1990;49(2): 231–41.
2. Pandozi C, Ficili S, Galeazzi M, et al. Propagation of the sinus impulse into the Koch triangle and localization, timing, and origin of the multicomponent potentials recorded in this area. Circ Arrhythm Electrophysiol 2011;4(2):225–34.
3. McGuire MA, Bourke JP, Robotin MC, et al. High resolution mapping of Koch's triangle using sixty electrodes in humans with atrioventricular junctional (AV nodal) reentrant tachycardia. Circulation 1993; 88(5 Pt 1):2315–28.
4. Li J, Greener ID, Inada S, et al. Computer three-dimensional reconstruction of the atrioventricular node. Circ Res 2008;102(8):975–85.
5. Mutharasan RK, Nagaraj A, Hamilton AJ, et al. Computer three-dimensional reconstruction of the atrioventricular conduction system. Pacing Clin Electrophysiol 2004;27(6 Pt 1):740–8.
6. Temple IP, Inada S, Dobrzynski H, et al. Connexins and the atrioventricular node. Heart Rhythm 2013; 10(2):297–304.
7. Frank M, Wirth A, Andrié RP, et al. Connexin45 provides optimal atrioventricular nodal conduction in the adult mouse heart. Circ Res 2012;111(12): 1528–38.
8. Ye Sheng X, Qu Y, Dan P, et al. Isolation and characterization of atrioventricular nodal cells from neonate rabbit heart. Circ Arrhythm Electrophysiol 2011;4(6): 936–46.
9. Greener ID, Monfredi O, Inada S, et al. Molecular architecture of the human specialised atrioventricular conduction axis. J Mol Cell Cardiol 2011;50(4): 642–51.
10. Dobrzynski H, Nikolski VP, Sambelashvili AT, et al. Site of origin and molecular substrate of atrioventricular junctional rhythm in the rabbit heart. Circ Res 2003;93(11):1102–10.
11. Goy JJ, Fromer M. Antiarrhythmic treatment of atrioventricular tachycardias. J Cardiovasc Pharmacol 1991;17(Suppl 6):S36–40.
12. Yamamoto M, Dobrzynski H, Tellez J, et al. Extended atrial conduction system characterised by the expression of the HCN4 channel and connexin45. Cardiovasc Res 2006;72(2):271–81.
13. Hucker WJ, McCain ML, Laughner JI, et al. Connexin 43 expression delineates two discrete

pathways in the human atrioventricular junction. Anat Rec (Hoboken) 2008;291(2):204–15.
14. Hucker WJ, Sharma V, Nikolski VP, et al. Atrioventricular conduction with and without AV nodal delay: two pathways to the bundle of His in the rabbit heart. Am J Physiol Heart Circ Physiol 2007;293(2):H1122–30.
15. Zhang Y, Bharati S, Mowrey KA, et al. His electrogram alternans reveal dual-wavefront inputs into and longitudinal dissociation within the bundle of His. Circulation 2001;104(7):832–8.
16. Greener ID, Tellez JO, Dobrzynski H, et al. Ion channel transcript expression at the rabbit atrioventricular conduction axis. Circ Arrhythm Electrophysiol 2009;2(3):305–15.
17. Zhang Y, Bharati S, Mowrey KA, et al. His electrogram alternans reveal dual atrioventricular nodal pathway conduction during atrial fibrillation: the role of slow-pathway modification. Circulation 2003; 107(7):1059–65.
18. Hucker WJ, Nikolski VP, Efimov IR. Autonomic control and innervation of the atrioventricular junctional pacemaker. Heart Rhythm 2007;4(10):1326–35.
19. Joung B, Tang L, Maruyama M, et al. Intracellular calcium dynamics and acceleration of sinus rhythm by beta-adrenergic stimulation. Circulation 2009; 119(6):788–96.
20. Zhang Y, Mazgalev TN. AV nodal dual pathway electrophysiology and Wenckebach periodicity. J Cardiovasc Electrophysiol 2011;22(11):1256–62.
21. Rosenblueth A. Mechanism of the Wenckebach-Luciani cycles. Am J Physiol 1958;194(3):491–4.
22. Hoshino K, Anumonwo J, Delmar M, et al. Wenckebach periodicity in single atrioventricular nodal cells from the rabbit heart. Circulation 1990;82(6):2201–16.
23. Efimov IR, Fahy GJ, Cheng Y, et al. High-resolution fluorescent imaging does not reveal a distinct atrioventricular nodal anterior input channel (fast pathway) in the rabbit heart during sinus rhythm. J Cardiovasc Electrophysiol 1997;8(3):295–306.
24. Efimov IR, Nikolski VP, Rothenberg F, et al. Structure-function relationship in the AV junction. Anat Rec A Discov Mol Cell Evol Biol 2004;280(2):952–65.
25. Hucker WJ, Fedorov VV, Foyil KV, et al. Images in cardiovascular medicine. Optical mapping of the human atrioventricular junction. Circulation 2008; 117(11):1474–7.
26. Fedorov VV, Ambrosi CM, Kostecki G, et al. Anatomic localization and autonomic modulation of atrioventricular junctional rhythm in failing human hearts. Circ Arrhythm Electrophysiol 2011;4(4): 515–25.
27. Arruda MS, McClelland JH, Wang X, et al. Development and validation of an ECG algorithm for identifying accessory pathway ablation site in Wolff-Parkinson-White syndrome. J Cardiovasc Electrophysiol 1998;9(1):2–12.

Arrhythmias Involving the Atrioventricular Junction

Luigi Di Biase, MD, PhD[a,b,c,d], Carola Gianni, MD, PhD[a],
Giuseppe Bagliani, MD[e,f,*], Luigi Padeletti, MD[g,h]

KEYWORDS

- Atrioventricular junction • Accessory pathway • Junctional tachycardia
- Atrioventricular node reentry tachycardia • Atrioventricular reentry tachycardia

KEY POINTS

- The atrioventricular junction is responsible for reentrant and automatic forms of supraventricular tachycardia.
- Atrioventricular nodal reentry tachycardia (AVNRT) is the most common supraventricular tachycardia, secondary to the presence of two electrophysiologically distinct pathways located near the atrioventricular node.
- Atrioventricular reentry tachycardia (AVRT) is more common in patients with ventricular preexcitation and is caused by the presence of an accessory pathway that bypasses the atrioventricular node.
- Junctional tachycardia (JT) is a rare form of nonparoxysmal supraventricular tachycardia, secondary to enhanced automaticity or triggered activity.
- There are many specific features that are seen on a simple 12-lead ECG hinting to the type of supraventricular tachycardia.

THE ATRIOVENTRICULAR JUNCTION

In normal sinus rhythm, the impulse travels from the sinus node to the ventricles following a craniocaudal direction. Along this path, there are relays that delay the conduction (ie, the atrioventricular node [AVN]) and systems that accelerate and optimize it (ie, the His-Purkinje system), usually preventing activation in the reverse order (from the ventricles to the atria). The atrioventricular (AV) junction is a complex structure that lies in the middle of this path, and consists of the compact AVN and surrounding structures (the AV nodal fibers and bundle of His before it branches). The AV junction has a central role in electrophysiology, responsible for reentrant and automatic forms of supraventricular tachycardia, AV nodal reentry tachycardia (AVNRT), and AV reentry tachycardia (AVRT), the most common tachycardias seen in the clinical setting, and junctional tachycardia (JT), which is discussed in this article.

No relevant conflicts to disclose.

[a] Texas Cardiac Arrhythmia Institute, St. David's Medical Center, 3000 N IH-35, Austin, TX, 78705, USA; [b] Department of Biomedical Engineering, University of Texas, 107 W Dean Keeton Street, Austin, TX, 78712, USA; [c] Arrhythmia Services, Montefiore Medical Center, Albert Einstein College of Medicine, 111 E 210th Street, Bronx, NY, 10467, USA; [d] Department of Clinical and Experimental Medicine, University of Foggia, Viale Pinto 1, 71122, Foggia (FG), Italy; [e] Arrhythmology Clinic Unit, Cardiology Department, Foligno General Hospital, Via Massimo Arcamone 5, 06034, Foligno (PG), Italy; [f] School of Cardiovascular Diseases, University of Perugia, Piazza Università 1, 06123, Perugia (PG), Italy; [g] Heart and Vessels Department, University of Florence, Largo Brambilla 3, 50134, Firenze (FI), Italy; [h] Cardiovascular Department IRCCS Multimedica, Sesto San Giovanni, Italy, Via Gaudenzio Fantoli, 16/15, 20138 Milano (MI), Italia
* Corresponding author. Arrhythmology Clinic Unit, Cardiology Department, Foligno General Hospital, Via Massimo Arcamone 5, 06034, Foligno (PG), Italy.
E-mail address: giuseppe.bagliani@tim.it

Card Electrophysiol Clin 9 (2017) 435–452
http://dx.doi.org/10.1016/j.ccep.2017.05.004

ATRIOVENTRICULAR NODAL REENTRY TACHYCARDIA

Electroanatomic Substrate

The AVN is located within the triangle of Koch, demarcated by the coronary sinus ostium, the tendon of Todaro, and the septal leaflet of the tricuspid valve.[1] The AVN is a highly specialized tissue that conducts slowly because its cells depolarize via slow inward calcium currents. The AVN is further divided into the compact node and its extensions, which connect it to the surrounding atrial tissue.[2] The compact AVN is usually located at the apex of the triangle of Koch, whereas its atrial connections extend inferiorly and posteriorly/superiorly. In 35% of the healthy population, these atrionodal connections possess distinct electrophysiologic properties: one connection has fast conduction velocity and a longer refractory period (the so-called, fast pathway), the other has slow conduction velocity but a shorter refractory period (slow pathway).[3,4] In the presence of a dual pathway, the normal sinus rhythm is mainly conducted via the fast pathway, which is more rapid (normal PR). However, when a premature atrial beat reaches the fast pathway when it is still refractory, the beat is conducted via the slow pathway (long PR). The phenomenon of selective anterograde conduction through the slow pathway (dual AVN physiology) is demonstrated by either the presence of two distinct PR intervals during normal sinus rhythm or an abrupt prolongation of the PR interval (at least 50 ms) after a small decrement (10 ms) of the premature impulse coupling interval ("jump"; **Fig. 1**).[5] However, a dual AVN physiology is not specific to patients with AVNRT, and two other events are necessary: the fast pathway has recovered by the time the impulse reaches the compact AVN, so that it be can conducted retrograde to the atria, producing an AVN echo beat (**Fig. 2**); and the echo beat is again conducted anterograde via the slow pathway, completing the circuit (*red arrow* in **Fig. 2**) and sustaining AVNRT (**Figs. 3** and **4**). This is the typical form of AVNRT, called slow-fast: the fast retrograde conduction leads the atria to depolarize almost synchronously with the ventricles, and the retrograde P wave on the electrocardiogram (ECG) is either hidden or only visible as a small deflection at the end of the QRS (*arrows* in **Figs. 4** and **5**). Less frequently, the circuit goes in the opposite direction, with the impulse traveling anterograde via the fast pathway and retrograde through the slow pathway.[6] This is the uncommon or atypical form of AVNRT (fast-slow): the atria depolarize long after the ventricles and the retrograde P wave on the ECG is late, close to the subsequent QRS (**Fig. 6**). Other rare variants AVNRT are described, and include slow-slow, fast-intermediate, and slow-intermediate forms in which two slow pathways, or one intermediate and fast or slow pathway are involved in reentry.[6,7] Usually, the cycle length is longer and the P wave is positioned clearly after the QRS (**Fig. 7**). The role of the atrial tissue in the reentry circuit remains controversial: in some cases, ventriculoatrial dissociation/block is observed (**Fig. 8**), indicating that the atrial tissue is not necessary in the reentry circuit. Similarly, the His bundle is a bystander: it is common to observe 2:1 AV block at the beginning of the tachycardia (**Fig. 9**).

Electrocardiogram

On the ECG, typical AVNRT is characterized by (1) a narrow QRS (unless aberrancy or pre-existing bundle branch block are present), (2) a regular

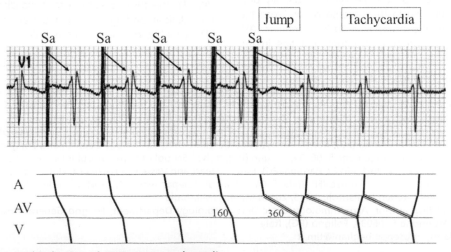

Fig. 1. Jump and induction of AVN reentry tachycardia.

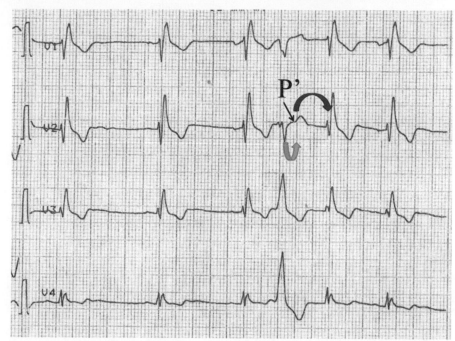

Fig. 2. AVN echo beat after a premature ventricular beat (*green arrow* shows fast pathway; *red arrow* shows slow pathway).

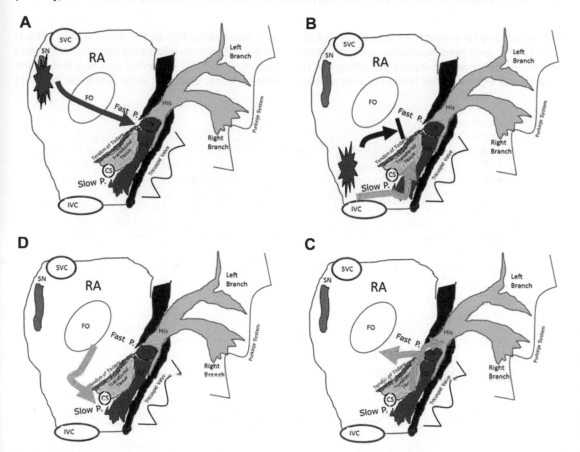

Fig. 3. Initiation of typical slow-fast AVNRT (see text for description). (*A*) Sinus beat. (*B*) Ectopic beat. (*C*) Echo beat. (*D*) AVNRT. CS, coronary sinus; CN, compact node; FO, fossa ovalis; INE, inferior nodal extension (slow pathway); IVC, inferior vena cava; RA, right atrium; SVC, superior vena cava.

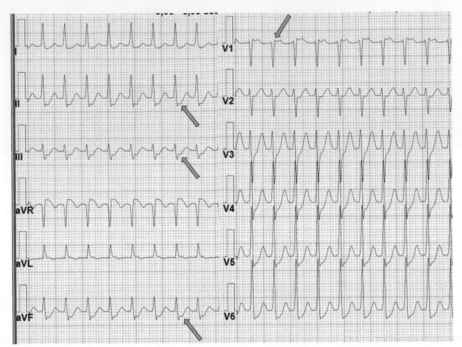

Fig. 4. Typical slow-fast AVNRT (*green arrows* show pseudo-S in the inferior leads and pseudo-R' in V1).

RR interval, and (3) a short RP (<70 ms). In typical AVNRT, the atria and ventricles are activated almost simultaneously, therefore the retrograde P wave on the ECG is either hidden or only visible as a small deflection at the end the QRS. The P wave in all rhythms originating from the AV junction (including AVNRT) is narrow and negative in the inferior leads, because atrial activation starts in

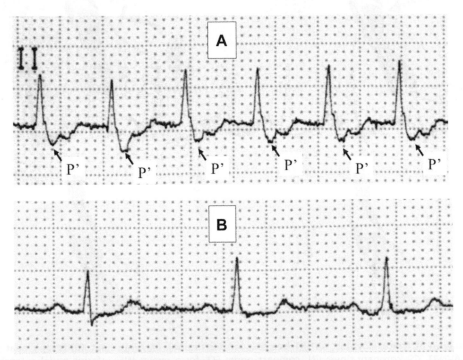

Fig. 5. (*A*) Pseudo-S1 in lead II during typical AVNRT. (*B*) Normal sinus rhythm.

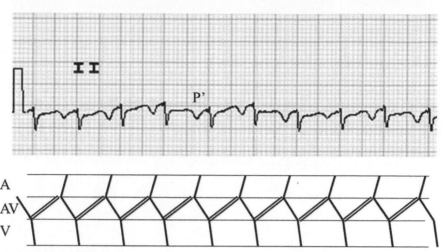

Fig. 6. Atypical fast-slow AVRT.

the low interatrial septum, spreading in a concentric and caudocranial fashion.

The P wave during typical AVNRT is difficult to see, and comparison with the ECG in normal sinus rhythm is especially useful (see **Fig. 5; Fig. 10**). When doing so, it is possible to spot the P wave as a pseudo-S wave in the inferior leads (see **Figs. 4, 5, 10; Fig. 11**) and/or a pseudo-R′ in V₁ (**Figs. 12** and **13**), mimicking an incomplete right bundle branch block (short RP). Identification of the P wave is not possible with pre-existing or functional bundle branch block because the P wave is simultaneous to the delayed components of the QRS (**Fig. 14**). The P wave is more easily recognized in atypical form of AVNRT, because it is located between the QRS, either early in the cycle (short RP, but >70 ms; slow-slow or fast/slow-intermediate forms, see **Fig. 7**) or late (long RP; fast-slow forms; see **Fig. 6; Fig. 15**). Ventricular repolarization is significantly affected by both the P wave (atrial depolarization) and atrial repolarization, mimicking myocardial ischemia even in normal hearts (**Fig. 16**).

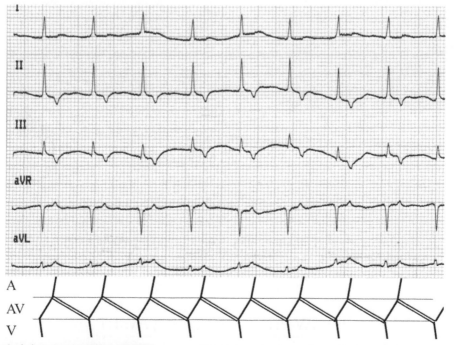

Fig. 7. Atypical slow-intermediate AVNRT.

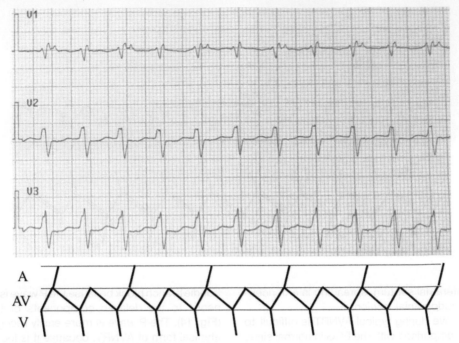

Fig. 8. A 2:1 VA conduction during AVNRT.

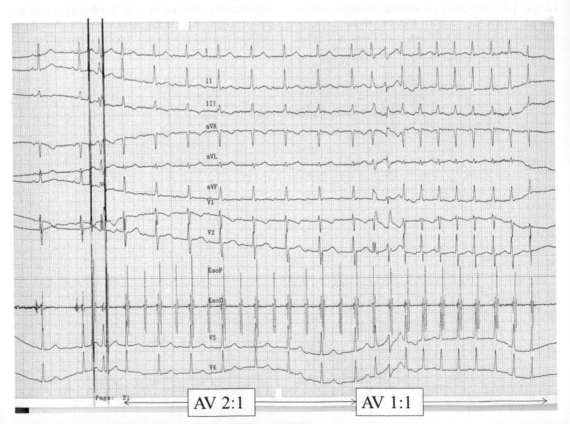

Fig. 9. Transient 2:1 AV conduction after induction of AVNRT.

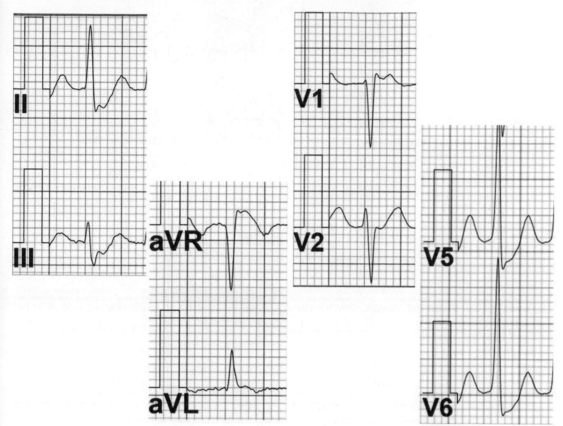

Fig. 10. Pseudo-S in the inferior leads and pseudo-R′ in V1 during typical slow-fast AVNRT.

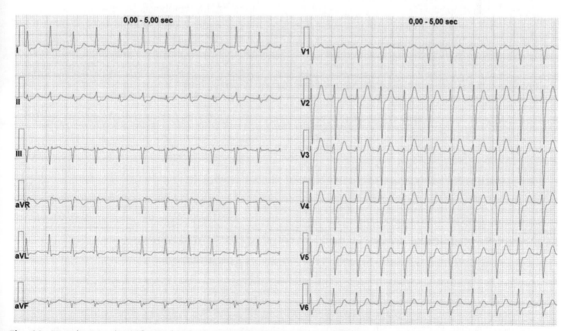

Fig. 11. Pseudo-S in the inferior leads during typical slow-fast AVNRT.

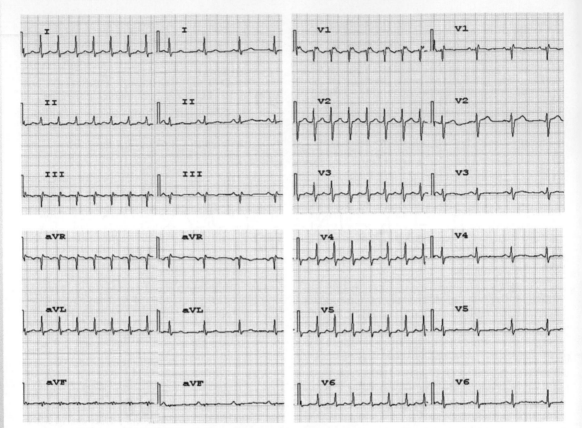

Fig. 12. Typical slow-fast AVNRT and sinus rhythm in the same patient.

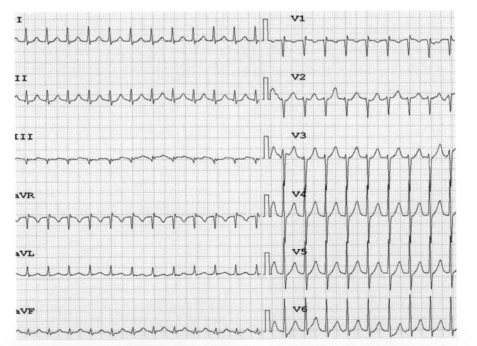

Fig. 13. Pseudo-R′ in V1 during typical slow-fast AVNRT.

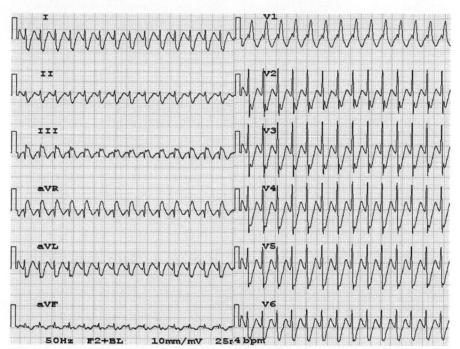

Fig. 14. Typical slow-fast AVNRT in a patient with pre-existing right bundle branch block.

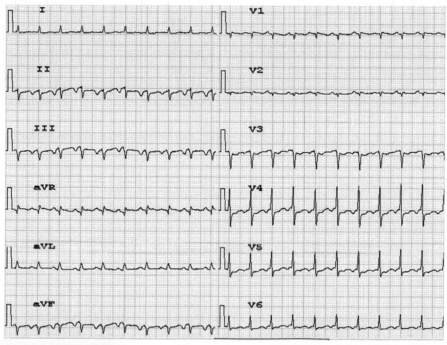

Fig. 15. Atypical fast-slow AVNRT.

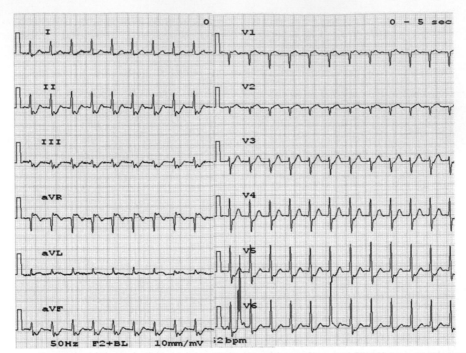

Fig. 16. Typical slow-fast AVNRT in a patient with repolarization changes mimicking myocardial ischemia.

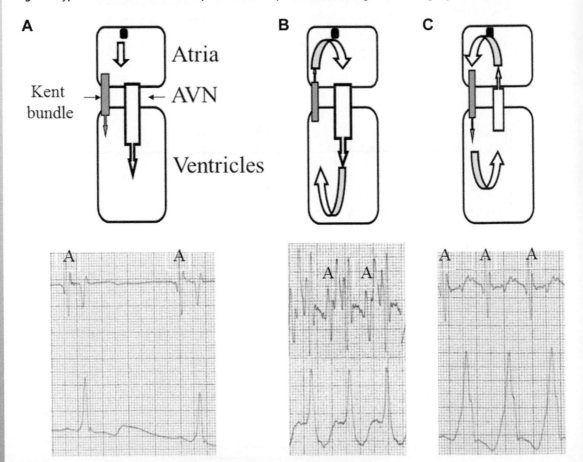

Fig. 17. Pre-excitation (*A*), orthodromic AVRT (*B*), and antidromic AVRT (*C*).

ATRIOVENTRICULAR REENTRY TACHYCARDIA
Electroanatomic Substrate

In the normal heart, the AV junction is the only connection between the atria and the ventricles. However, in some individuals, there are additional muscle bundles that connect the atria and the ventricles, allowing electrical impulses to bypass the AV junction, the so-called AV accessory pathways (AP) or bypass tracts, located essentially anywhere around the AV groove.[8] In contrast to the AVN, APs usually conduct rapidly, because they are comprised of myocardial cells that depolarize via the fast sodium current. Most of the APs can conduct in an anterograde and retrograde fashion: the ECG is characteristic, with a short PR and ventricular pre-excitation (delta wave). However, some APs are only capable of conduction in one direction, usually retrograde (concealed APs). In this case, the ECG is normal but the AP can still participate in the circuit of AVRT. AVRT is a macro-reentrant tachycardia, in which the atria and ventricles are activated sequentially, using two distinct pathways, the AV junction and the AP (**Fig. 17**A). The circuit of AVRT can rotate in two directions: in one, the impulse activates the ventricles through the normal AV junction–Purkinje system, generating a normal QRS (orthodromic AVRT; see **Fig. 17**B); in the other, the impulse activates the ventricles through the AP, and the QRS is wide (antidromic AVRT; see **Fig. 17**C). As in AVNRT, a premature beat along with the differential electrophysiologic properties of the involved pathways (more specifically, the AP has a longer refractory period compared with the AVN) are key to initiate AVRT (**Fig. 18**). In orthodromic AVRT, a premature atrial beat reaches the AP when it is still refractory, and is conducted to the ventricles exclusively through AV junction. For manifest AP, this leads to the disappearance of ventricular pre-excitation and normalization of the PR interval. After depolarization of the ventricles, the impulse is conducted retrograde though the AP, producing an atrial echo beat. If this AVN is excitable, the impulse is again conducted anterograde via the AV junction, the circuit completes, and AVRT sustains. Because the atria and the ventricles are activated sequentially, the P wave falls after the QRS (**Fig. 19**). Orthodromic AVRT can also be easily induced by a premature ventricular

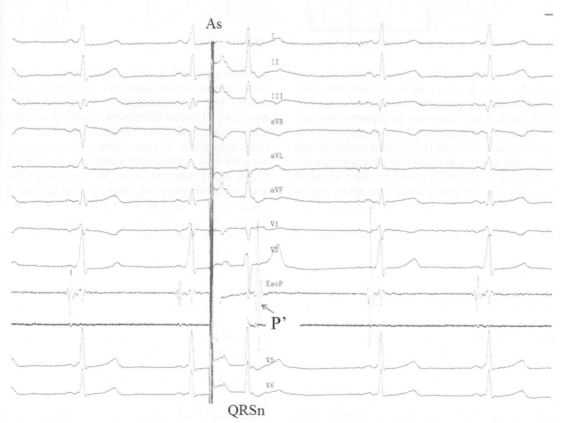

Fig. 18. Atrioventricular "echo" beat after a single premature atrial stimulation (As): PR interval prolongs, QRS normalizes (QRSn); an atrial echo beat (P') is well evident at esophageal recording.

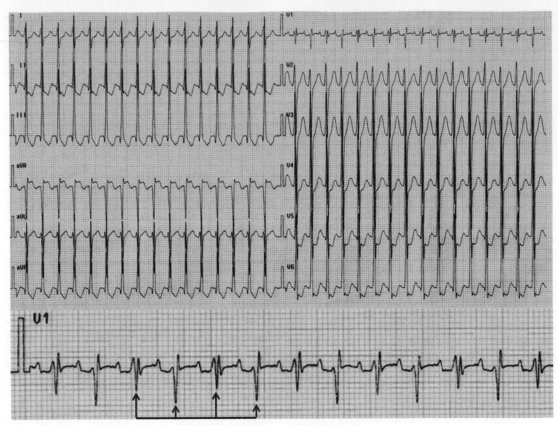

Fig. 19. Atrioventricular reentry tachycardia (*arrows* show QRS alternans).

beat, and it is typical for concealed APs: the impulse finds the distal conduction system refractory and is retrograde conducted to the atria via the AP. Conversely, it is uncommon for a premature ventricular beat to induce AVNRT, because it requires the impulse to find the His-Purkinje nonrefractory to be able to enter the AVN and initiate the tachycardia. Antidromic AVRT is less common, because it requires an AP with a shorter refractory period than the AVN: this is usually true in patients with AVN disease or when the premature beat originates close or within an AP that is located far from the AVN (**Fig. 20**). The premature impulse activates the ventricles via the AP and is retroconducted via the AV junction, activating the atria again and completing the circuit. Not infrequently, antidromic AVRTs use a second AP as the retrograde limb. Because the ventricles are activated via the AP, the ECG is maximally pre-excited and it is difficult to visualize the P wave (**Fig. 21**).

Atypical Accessory Pathways

Although APs usually connect the atria and the ventricle with fast conduction properties, there are some exceptions.[9] More specifically, there is a peculiar concealed AP, with slow conduction

properties (AVN-like) and usually located in the posteroseptal region, close to the coronary sinus ostium. This is responsible for a form of orthodromic AVRT called permanent junctional reciprocating tachycardia (PJRT) or Coumel tachycardia. This tachycardia is characteristically incessant, because it can initiate with a simple sinus impulse that is easily retroconducted to the atria via the slow AP, leading to a very long RP (**Fig. 22**). Other rare atypical variants of APs connect (1) atrium to the AVN (atrionodal), the His (atriohisian), or the fascicles (atriofascicular); (2) the node to the fascicles (nodofascicular) or the ventricle (nodoventricular); or (3) the fascicle to the ventricles (fasciculoventricular). The most common form of AVRT involving an atypical AP is the so-called Mahaim tachycardia, an antidromic AVRT using a long anterograde-only atriofascicular pathway that connects the right atrial free wall to the distal part of the right bundle. As such, the ECG during the tachycardia is pre-excited, with a left bundle branch block morphology (**Fig. 23**).

Electrocardiogram

On the ECG (see **Fig. 19**), orthodromic AVRT is characterized by (1) a narrow QRS (unless

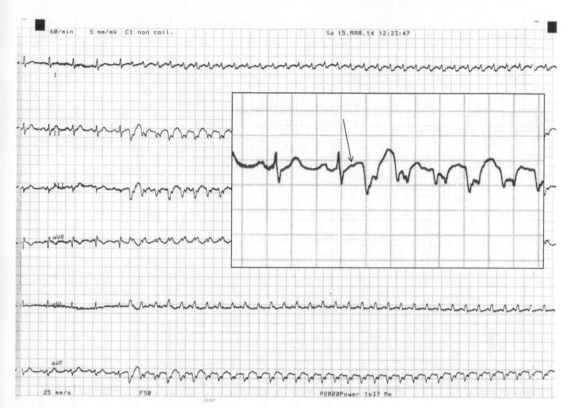

Fig. 20. Initiation of antidromic AVRT by a premature atrial beat (*arrow*).

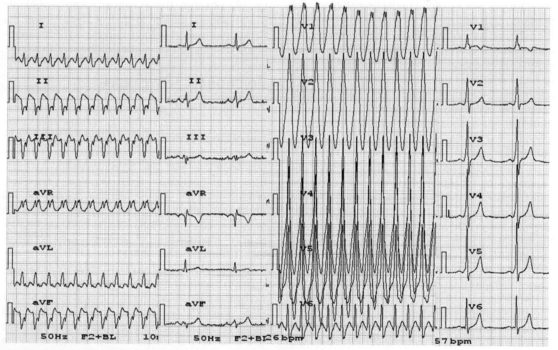

Fig. 21. Antidromic AVRT and sinus rhythm in the same patient.

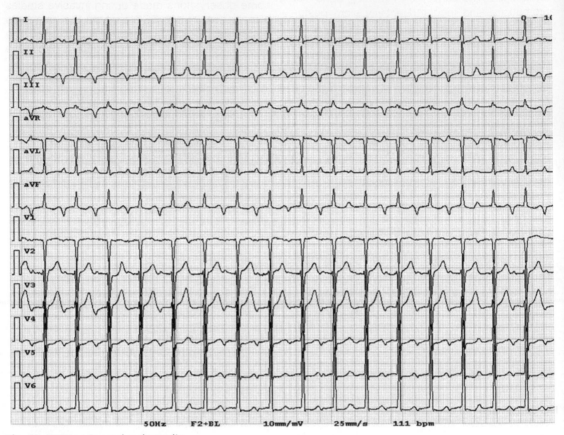

Fig. 22. PJRT or Coumel tachycardia.

aberrancy or pre-existing bundle branch block are present), (2) a regular RR interval, and (3) a short RP (>70 ms; except for PJRT). An interesting phenomenon that is commonly (up to 30%) observed in AVRT is electrical alternans of the QRS, a beat-to-beat variation of the QRS amplitude. The mechanism of QRS alternans is not clear, but is commonly observed when the rate is very rapid; therefore, it is speculated that it results from oscillations in the relative refractory period of the distal conduction system. In orthodromic AVRT, the P wave morphology is variable, and it mostly depends on the location of the APs: with septal or paraseptal APs, the P wave is similar to that of AVNRT (narrow, negative in the inferior leads, and positive in aVL and aVR); with APs located in the left free wall the P wave is negative in lead I, aVL, and V_4 to V_6 (apical leads), whereas in right-sided APs, the P wave is negative in V_1 and positive in lead I, aVL, and V_4 to V_6.

The ECG during antidromic AVRTs (see **Figs. 20** and **21**) is characterized by (1) a wide QRS (secondary to maximal pre-excitation), (2) a regular RR interval, and (3) a variable RP (if short, >70 ms). The width of the QRS and the ST-T segment

usually obscure the P wave; when visible, its morphology is similar to that of AVNRT, and the RP interval is short or long, depending on the retrograde conduction properties of the AV junction.

JUNCTIONAL TACHYCARDIA

The cells in the AV junction are capable of spontaneous depolarization. This is usually lower than that of the sinus node, and it allows the AV junction to operate as a subsidiary pacemaker when the sinus node fails (**Fig. 24**). Sometimes, the AV junction can generate rapid impulses, therefore producing a JT. This is usually caused by the enhanced automaticity in the setting of ischemia or inflammation (eg, following cardiac surgery), or delayed afterdepolarizations in the setting of digitalis toxicity.[10] The exact site of origin of this rhythm is unclear, although by observing the relationship between the P and the QRS one can hypothesize that (1) when the P wave precedes the QRS (**Fig. 25**) the site is above the compact node, (2) when the P wave is within the QRS the site is within the compact AVN, and (3) when the P wave is after the QRS (**Fig. 26**) the site is below

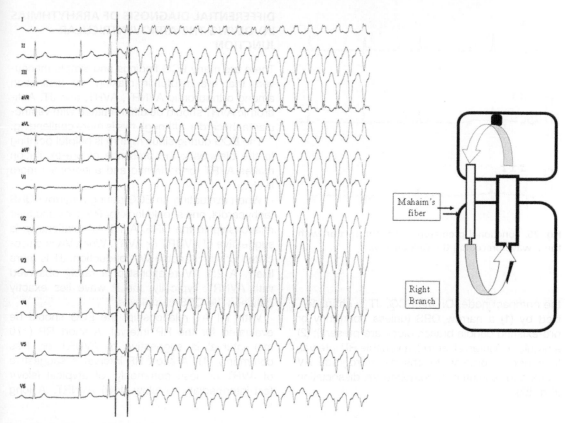

Fig. 23. Mahaim tachycardia.

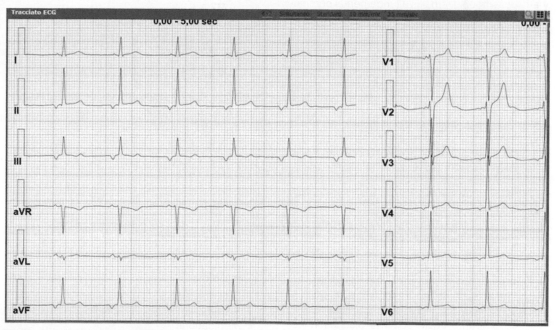

Fig. 24. Junctional escape rhythm.

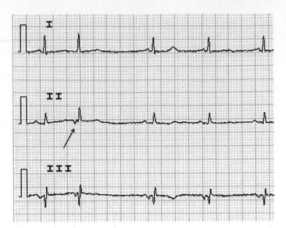

Fig. 25. Junctional premature atrial contraction with the P wave preceding the QRS (*arrow*).

the compact node. On the ECG, JT is characterized by (1) a narrow QRS (unless aberrancy or pre-existing bundle branch block are present); (2) a regular RR interval; and (3) a variable RP interval. It is not uncommon to observe retrograde AV block and, sometimes, complete VA dissociation (**Fig. 27**).

DIFFERENTIAL DIAGNOSIS OF ARRHYTHMIAS INVOLVING THE ATRIOVENTRICULAR JUNCTION

There are many ECG findings and simple maneuvers that are helpful in making the distinction among orthodromic AVNRT, AVRT, and JT. Antidromic AVRT should be differentiated with ventricular tachycardia, although this is more challenging.

The ECG during sinus rhythm is helpful pointing to the diagnosis: the presence of pre-excitation makes AVRT (orthodromic and antidromic) more likely.

When evaluating an ECG during a narrow-QRS tachycardia, one should look for P waves and their relationship to the QRS. A 1:1 AV relationship is suggestive of AVNRT or AVRT. When VA is dissociated or with variable VA conduction, JT is more likely. A 2:1 AV relationship is rarely observed with AVNRT: typically, the P wave lies exactly between the QRS complexes.

With 1:1 AV relationship, the ECG should be evaluated for the RP interval. A short RP (<70 ms) interval is suggestive of AVNRT or, less commonly, JT. A short RP interval is suggestive of AVRT or, less commonly, of atypical (slow/fast-intermediate or slow-slow) AVNRT. A long

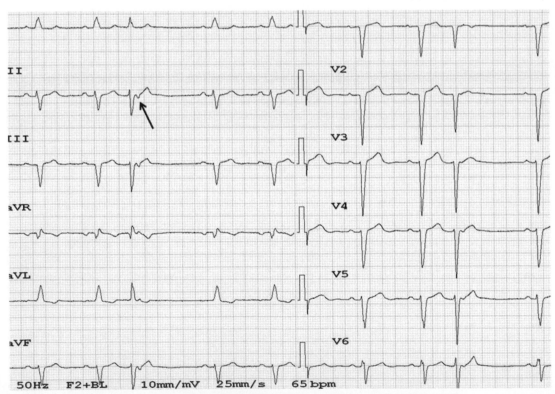

Fig. 26. Junctional premature atrial contraction with the P wave following the QRS (*arrow*).

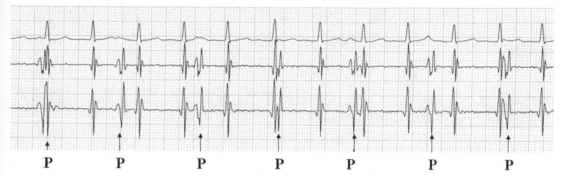

Fig. 27. Ventriculoatrial dissociation during junctional tachycardia (P waves in the esophageal recordings).

RP interval is suggestive of PJRT, atypical (fast-slow) AVNRT, or JT.

The P wave morphology when discernible can help. A narrow, superiorly direct P wave is typical of AVNRT, orthodromic AVNRT involving a septal AP, or JT.

As for the QRS, there two important clues. First, the presence of QRS alternans is more common in AVRT, but is also seen in fast AVNRT. Second, if a bundle branch block develops during the tachy-cardia, a slowing of the tachycardia rate with bundle branch block is diagnostic of AVRT using an AP on the same side as the blocked branch (Coumel law; **Fig. 28**); when both right bundle branch block and left bundle branch block are present, the APs are located on the same side as the branch associated with the longest RR interval when blocked (**Fig. 29**).

Finally, the mode of initiation and termination is helpful. Initiation after a single premature atrial beat with a marked prolongation of the PR is typical of AVNRT. Initiation and termination after a single premature ventricular beat are suggestive of AVRT.

Recurrent initiation without a premature beat is characteristic of PJRT. A gradual acceleration (warm-up phenomenon) is typical of automatic rhythms, therefore suggesting JT. Termination with vagal maneuvers or adenosine is typical of AVRT or AVNRT, whereas JT (and VT) continues with VA block.

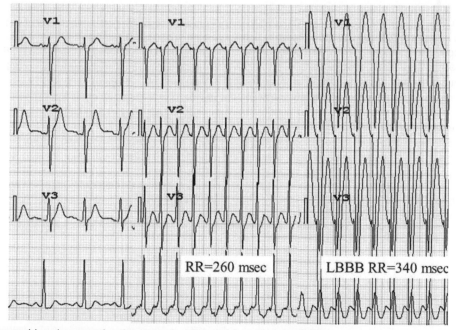

Fig. 28. Coumel law (see text for description). LBBB, left bundle branch block.

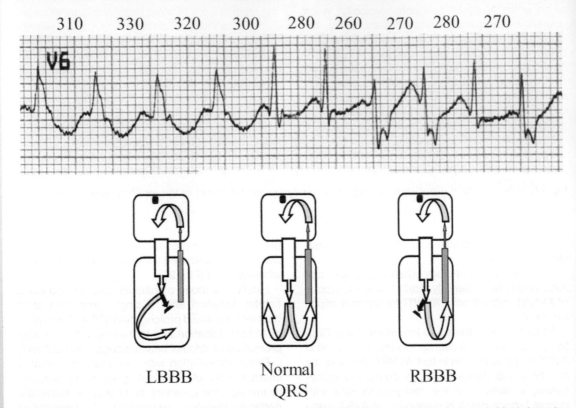

Fig. 29. Coumel law in a patient with right bundle branch block (RBBB) and left bundle branch block (LBBB).

REFERENCES

1. Sánchez-Quintana D, Yen Ho S. Anatomy of cardiac nodes and atrioventricular specialized conduction system. Rev Esp Cardiol 2003;56(11):1085–92.

2. Kurian T, Ambrosi C, Hucker W, et al. Anatomy and electrophysiology of the human AV node. Pacing Clin Electrophysiol 2010;33(6):754–62.

3. Medkour D, Becker AE, Khalife K, et al. Anatomic and functional characteristics of a slow posterior AV nodal pathway: role in dual-pathway physiology and reentry. Circulation 1998;98(2):164–74.

4. Mani BC, Pavri BB. Dual atrioventricular nodal pathways physiology: a review of relevant anatomy, electrophysiology, and electrocardiographic manifestations. Indian Pacing Electrophysiol J 2014; 14(1):12–25.

5. Brooks R, Goldberger J, Kadish A. Extended protocol for demonstration of dual AV nodal physiology. Pacing Clin Electrophysiol 1993;16(2):277–84.

6. Heidbüchel H, Jackman WM. Characterization of subforms of AV nodal reentrant tachycardia. Europace 2004;6(4):316–29.

7. Katritsis DG, Camm AJ. Classification and differential diagnosis of atrioventricular nodal re-entrant tachycardia. Europace 2006;8(1):29.

8. Ho SY. Accessory atrioventricular pathways. Circulation 2008;117(12):1502–4.

9. Issa ZF, Miller JM, Zipes DP. Variants of preexcitation. In: Clinical arrhythmology and electrophysiology. 2nd edition. Amsterdam: Elsevier; 2012. p. 468–79.

10. Liu CF, Ip JE, Lin AC, et al. Mechanistic heterogeneity of junctional ectopic tachycardia in adults. Pacing Clin Electrophysiol 2013;36(1):e7–10.

The QRS Complex
Normal Activation of the Ventricles

Giuseppe Bagliani, MD[a,b,*], Roberto De Ponti, MD, FHRS[c], Carola Gianni, MD, PhD[d], Luigi Padeletti, MD[e,f]

KEYWORDS

- QRS complex • Ventricular conduction system • Bundle branch block • Ashman phenomenon

KEY POINTS

- The ventricular conduction comprises the right and left bundle branches and the Purkinje network.
- The ventricular conduction system is responsible for the synchronized and almost simultaneous activation of both ventricles.
- The QRS complex is determined by the electrical currents originating from ventricular depolarization.
- Any change in the normal ventricular activation sequence determines a delay that produces a wide QRS on the surface electrocardiogram, usually secondary to delay or block in one of the 2 branches.
- The Ashman phenomenon is a kind of functional aberrant conduction that occurs after a long-short cycle.

INTRODUCTION

The currents generated by ventricular depolarization (when transmitted to the body surface) generate the QRS complex, a sequence of high-amplitude waves visible on the 12-lead electrocardiogram (ECG). The well-ordered sequence of the QRS waves is caused by the synchronized electrical activation of the myocardium driven by the ventricular conduction system. The primary function of the ventricular conduction system is to synchronize the segmental activation of the ventricles, optimizing energy demand. In a normal heart, the ventricular contraction starts at the apex of the heart and moves with a twisting motion to the side walls, reaching the base of the heart, ensuring that blood is directed toward the outflow tracts of the 2 ventricles using the least amount of energy.

THE VENTRICULAR CONDUCTION SYSTEM

The ventricular conduction system starts below the His bundle, where it bifurcates into the 2 bundle branches (right and left) that taper out to the subendocardial Purkinje network, which in turn activates the ventricular myocardium. Although the bundle of His divides into 2 branches, it is normal to consider the ventricular conduction as a trifascicular system, because the left bundle branch subdivides into 2 fascicles (anterior and posterior), which are anatomically distinct and activate the left ventricle simultaneously from 2 areas, optimizing the ventricular contraction. In contrast,

Disclosure: The authors have no relevant conflicts to disclose.
[a] Arrhythmology Unit, Cardiology Department, Foligno General Hospital, Via Massimo Arcamone, 06034 Foligno (PG), Italy; [b] Cardiovascular Diseases Department, University of Perugia, Piazza Menghini 1, 06129 Perugia, Italy; [c] Cardiology Department, University of Insubria, Via Ravasi, 2, 21100 Varese, Italy; [d] Texas Cardiac Arrhythmia Institute, St. David's Medical Center, 3000 N IH 35, Ste 700, Austin, TX 78705, USA; [e] Heart and Vessels Department, University of Florence, Largo Brambilla, 3, 50134 Florence, Italy; [f] IRCCS Multimedica, Cardiology Department, Via Milanese, 300, 20099 Sesto San Giovanni, Italy
* Corresponding author. Cardiovascular Diseases Department, University of Perugia, Piazza Menghini 1, 06129 Perugia, Italy.
E-mail address: giuseppe.bagliani@tim.it

Card Electrophysiol Clin 9 (2017) 453–460
http://dx.doi.org/10.1016/j.ccep.2017.05.005
1877-9182/17/© 2017 Elsevier Inc. All rights reserved.

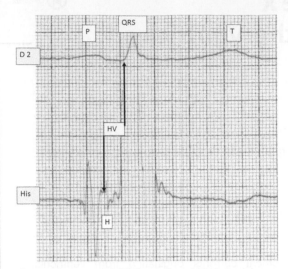

Fig. 1. His potential (H) (*arrow*) and HV interval.

the right bundle branch does not have functionally or anatomically distinguishable pathways and it is considered a single fascicle. The trifascicular system activates the Purkinje network, a subendocardial plexiform layer of dense intramural branches able to finely activate the small corresponding segmental myocardial segments. For this reason, under normal conditions, the myocardium is activated from the endocardium toward the epicardium.

The electrical activation of the ventricular conduction system produces very low amplitude currents that cannot be detected on the surface ECG, and the QRS comprises electrical currents originating from the contractile myocardium. Activation of the ventricular conduction system lies in the

terminal portion of the PR interval, and can be detected only by intracardiac recordings: electrodes positioned at the level of the atrioventricular junction can record activation of the His bundle (His potential; **Fig. 1**), and the interval between the recording of His bundle electrogram and the beginning of the QRS (the so-called HV interval) represents the activation of the ventricular conduction system.

THE NORMAL QRS

The QRS complex represents ventricular depolarization, the electrical activation of the myocardial mass. Normal ventricular depolarization is a rapid process, and the subsequent QRS complex comprises electrical signals of high amplitude and steep slope, with a duration between 80 and 110 milliseconds. The nomenclature of the QRS refers to the sequence of deflections seen in lead I: the Q wave is the first negative wave placed at the beginning of the QRS, the R wave is the first positive deflection, whereas the S wave is the terminal negative deflection. Activation of the various ventricular myocardium segments does not take place simultaneously but according to a precise temporal sequence such as that depolarization starts from the apical portion of the interventricular septum and continues toward the side walls up to the base of the ventricles. This complex process of activation determines 3 successive activation fronts, each represented by a distinct electric vector, contributing to the overall morphology of the QRS complex (**Fig. 2**):

- The first vector (activation of the apical portion of the interventricular septum) is directed from left to right, has a duration of less than

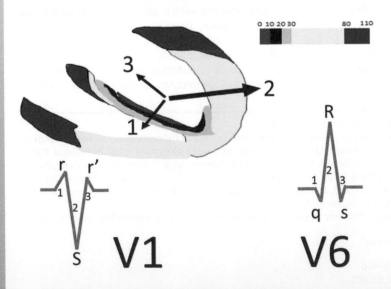

Fig. 2. Vectorial determinants of the QRS complex.

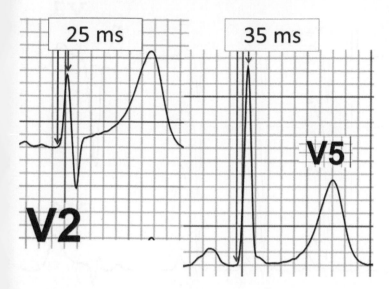

Fig. 3. Intrinsicoid deflection in the right and left precordial leads.

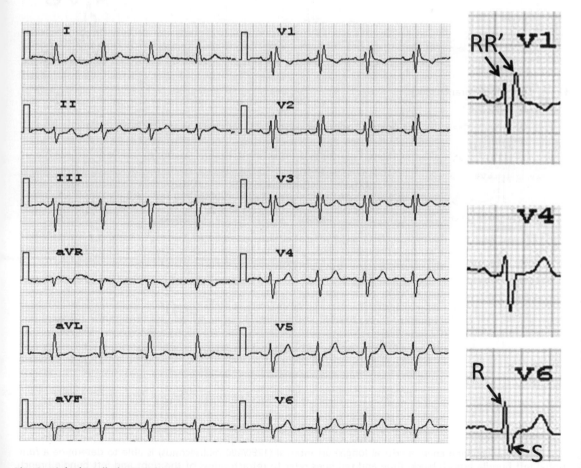

Fig. 4. Right bundle branch block.

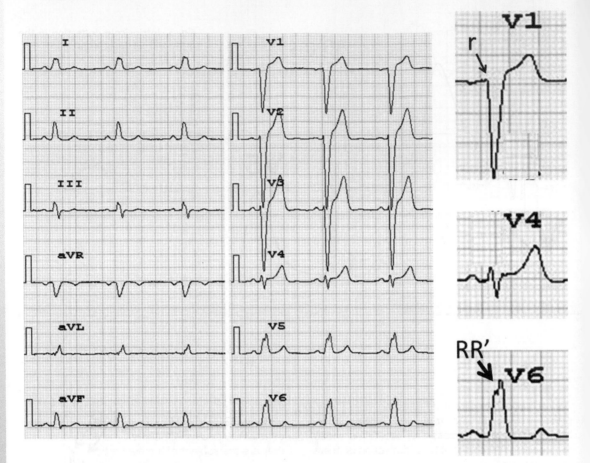

Fig. 5. Left bundle branch block.

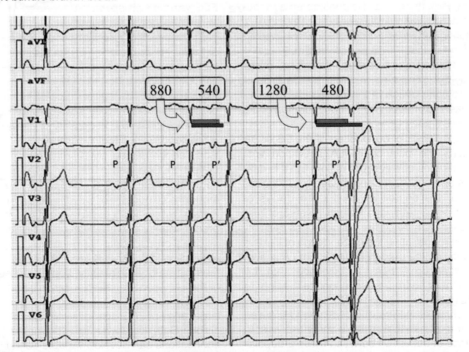

Fig. 6. Ashman phenomenon: a critical long/short interval (1280/480 milliseconds) is able to determine a functional left bundle branch block. Blue and red lines refer to refractoriness of the right and left bundle branch, respectively, which varies according to the previous cycle length.

40 milliseconds with an amplitude of less than one-third of the total QRS amplitude, and forms the small Q wave in the left ventricular leads (I, aVL, V5 and V6) and the small initial R in the right precordial leads (V1 and V2)

- The second vector (activation of the large left ventricular mass) is the dominant part of ventricular activation, directed down and to the left, and is responsible for the broad R wave that is usually recorded in the left ventricular leads and the negative S wave of the right precordial leads
- The third vector (activation of the right ventricle and basal portions of the left ventricle and interventricular septum) is directed upward and to the right, determining the small S wave recorded in the left ventricular leads and the small terminal R wave sometimes visible in the right precordial leads

INTRINSICOID DEFLECTION

The intrinsicoid deflection (or R wave peak time) is the time between the onset of Q or R wave and the peak of the R wave in the left ventricular lateral leads, and it represents the time taken for ventricular activation to spread from the endocardium to the epicardium. More specifically, under normal conditions, the intrinsicoid deflection expresses the time required for local intramural activation of the directly explored myocardium: for this reason, it should be calculated only in the precordial leads (which record the electrical activity of the myocardial wall directly below the exploring electrode) and not in the peripheral leads, which do not explore specific segments of the myocardium but the whole electrical activity of the heart. The intrinsicoid deflection of the right precordial leads, exploring thinner myocardial areas, has a shorter duration than that of the left precordial leads (**Fig. 3**): as such, the normal duration of the intrinsicoid deflection in leads V1 and V2 is less than 35 milliseconds, whereas in V5 and V6 it is less than 45 milliseconds.

A prolonged intrinsicoid deflection represents conditions for an increased time for the ventricular activation to spread from the endocardium to the epicardium, such as left ventricular

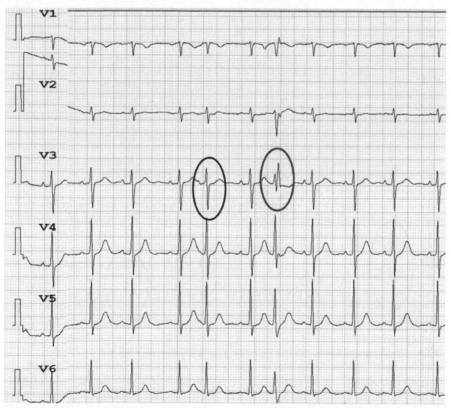

Fig. 7. Functional right bundle branch block. Two premature atrial beats: the first is normally conducted (*black circle*) and the second shows a functional right branch block (*red circle*) caused by a critical long/short interval.

hypertrophy, interventricular conduction delay, and ventricular ectopic beats. A careful analysis of the intrinsicoid deflection can be useful to differentiate between a wide QRS secondary to a conduction disease or with an ectopic origin (See article by Roberto De Ponti and colleagues', article "General approach to a wide QRS complex," in this issue).

FUNCTIONAL AND ANATOMIC BUNDLE BRANCH BLOCK

Any change in the aforementioned ventricular activation sequence determines a delay that produces a wide QRS (duration ≥120 milliseconds) on the surface ECG. When a branch does not conduct normally (with either delay or block), the Purkinje network of the ipsilateral ventricle is depolarized late, by the front coming from the contralateral ventricle. The QRS of a bundle branch block is characteristic, with a morphology that depends on the blocked branch/fascicle (**Figs. 4** and **5**).

Right Bundle Branch Block

In the presence of right bundle branch block, the initial septal activation (first vector) and the activation of the left ventricle (second vector) are unchanged, whereas the late activation of the right ventricle forces the third vector to prolong, with the characteristic triphasic ECG pattern constituted by a second R wave (R'), evident in the right

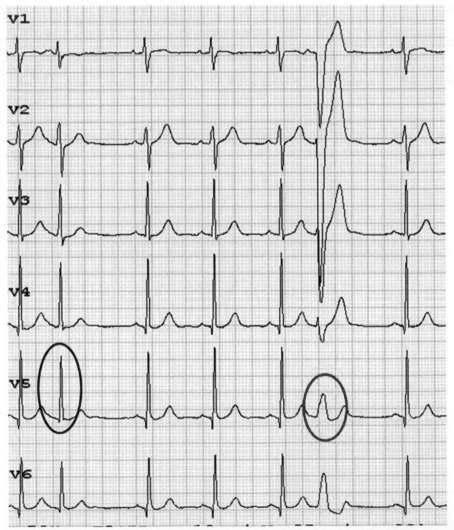

Fig. 8. Functional left bundle branch block. Two premature atrial beats: the first is normally conducted (*black circle*) and the second, after a critical long/short interval, shows a functional left bundle branch block (*red circle*).

precordial leads (see **Fig. 4**), which show a prolonged intrinsicoid deflection. In the left precordial leads, the late right ventricular activation is shown by the presence of a wide S wave (usually ≥40 milliseconds).

Left Bundle Branch Block

In the presence of left bundle branch block, the first vector, which depends on the activation of the Purkinje network in the left portion of the interventricular septum, is inverted or seriously compromised and both Q wave in the left leads and R wave in the right leads decrease or disappear (**Fig. 5**). The second ventricular activation vector is longer because of the delayed depolarization of the left ventricle that occurs after the right ventricular activation is completed. The QRS complex is therefore composed of a monophasic positive complex in the left precordial leads and a monophasic negative complex in right precordial leads; accordingly, the left-sided intrinsicoid deflection is clearly delayed.

Bundle branch blocks can be secondary to a primitive conduction disease or to a functional conduction delay. In the former, there is an anatomic reason for the block/delay, whereas the latter occurs when there is a change in the heart rate and depends on the different durations of the refractory period of the two branches.[1] The most common form of functional conduction delay is the Ashman phenomenon, a kind of aberrant conduction that occurs after a long-short cycle (**Fig. 6**).[2] The branches are composed of sodium-dependent cells, and their refractory period depends on the length of the previous cardiac cycle: the longer the cycle, the greater the refractory period, and therefore the greater the likelihood of branch conduction block in case of a subsequent premature atrial beat. Of note, a functional right bundle branch block pattern (**Fig. 7**) is more common than a left bundle branch block (**Fig. 8**) pattern because of the longer refractory period of the right bundle. In rare cases, the ventricular complexes remain wide after the initial aberrancy, because of continuous retrograde concealed conduction into the anterogradely blocked branch, which will be refractory for the next oncoming supraventricular impulse (linking phenomenon; See article by Roberto De Ponti and colleagues', article "General approach to a wide QRS complex," in this issue).[3] This persisting aberrancy usually resolves after a sufficiently long cycle which allows the supraventricular impulse to reach both branches outside after their

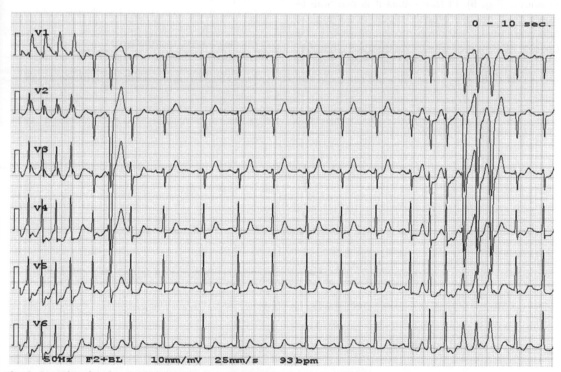

Fig. 9. Functional right and left bundle branch block in the same patient.

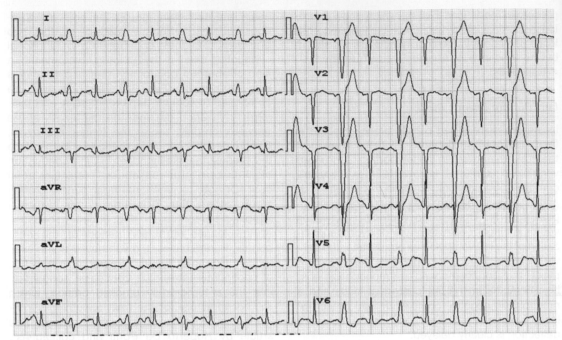

Fig. 10. Alternating left bundle branch block.

refractory period (reverse Ashman phenomenon) following a short-long cycle. Given the functionality of the mechanisms that are the basis of the phenomenon, it is possible to observe in the same patient both left and right branch block aberrances (**Fig. 9**). In rare cases it is possible to observe a bundle branch block occurring on alternate beats; although more frequent in the case of alternating RR interval duration, the phenomenon can also be evident with a constant sinus cycle (**Fig. 10**).

REFERENCES

1. Denker S, Shenasa M, Gilbert CJ, et al. Effects of abrupt changes in cycle length on refractoriness of the His-Purkinje system in man. Circulation 1983; 67(1):60–8.
2. Gouaux JL, Ashman R. Auricular fibrillation with aberration simulating ventricular paroxysmal tachycardia. Am Heart J 1947;34(3):366–73.
3. Lehmann MH, Denker S, Mahmud R, et al. Linking: a dynamic electrophysiologic phenomenon in macro-reentry circuits. Circulation 1985;71(2):254–65.

General Approach to a Wide QRS Complex

Roberto De Ponti, MD, FHRS[a], Giuseppe Bagliani, MD[b,c,*], Luigi Padeletti, MD[d,e], Andrea Natale, MD, FACC, FHRS, FESC[f,g,h,i,j]

KEYWORDS

- QRS complex • Wide complex tachycardia • Ventricular tachycardia • Supraventricular tachycardia
- Aberrancy

KEY POINTS

- A wide QRS complex (≥120 ms) is present when the normal activation pattern (His–bundle branches–Purkinje) is modified.
- It is important to differentiate between ventricular tachycardia and supraventricular tachycardia conducted with aberrancy because this significantly influences the management.
- The presence of ventriculoatrial dissociation (either by identifying dissociated atrial activity or noting capture and fusion beats) is the most helpful electrocardiographic sign of ventricular tachycardia.
- The Brugada and Vereckei algorithms, which use a combination of ventriculoatrial dissociation and QRS morphology criteria, are commonly used for the differential diagnosis of wide QRS tachycardia.
- All the conditions modifying structurally the activation of the heart (pacemakers, ventricular preexcitation, severe myocardial disease, hyperkaliemia, antiarrhythmic or psychotropic drugs) should be known to provide a precise differential diagnosis of a wide QRS.

INTRODUCTION

The term "wide QRS complex" is generally used as an electrocardiographic (ECG) jargon in the presence of a QRS complex with increased duration, greater than or equal to 120 milliseconds. Although "wide QRS complex" frequently refers to a wide complex tachycardia (WCT), a wide QRS complex is present also in a single beat, and during bradycardia. Because duration is the only discriminant, it should be accurately measured on a standard 12-lead ECG, from the onset of the QRS complex to its terminal components. Indeed, measurement of the QRS duration in a single lead may frequently result in an inaccurate evaluation and, therefore, it should be avoided. The approach to an ECG showing wide QRS complexes frequently represents a great challenge in clinical practice. Wide QRS complex results from a variety of mechanisms and clinical conditions and its correct interpretation is crucial for differential diagnosis and appropriate decision making.

CAUSES OF A WIDE QRS COMPLEX

Narrow QRS complex is the ECG equivalent of a well-defined, ordered, and reproducible activation sequence of both ventricles through the His

No relevant conflicts to disclose.
[a] Cardiology Department, University of Insubria, Varese, Italy; [b] Arrhythmology Unit, Cardiology Department, Foligno General Hospital, Foligno, Italy; [c] Cardiovascular Diseases Department, University of Perugia, Perugia, Italy; [d] Heart and Vessels Department, University of Florence, Florence, Italy; [e] IRCCS Multimedica, Sesto San Giovanni, Italy, [f] Texas Cardiac Arrhythmia Institute, St. David's Medical Center, Austin, TX, USA; [g] Doll Medical School, University of Texas, Austin, TX, USA; [h] MetroHealth Medical Center, Case Western Reserve University School of Medicine, Cleveland, OH, USA; [i] Division of Cardiology, Stanford University, Stanford, CA, USA; [j] Electrophysiology and Arrhythmia Services, California Pacific Medical Center, San Francisco, CA, USA
* Corresponding author. Arrhythmology Unit, Cardiology Department, Foligno General Hospital, Foligno, Italy.
E-mail address: giuseppe.bagliani@tim.it

bundle, bundle branches, and Purkinje network. Every event that modifies this sequence results in QRS prolongation. More specifically, a wide QRS can be seen in the presence of the following causes:

- Ectopic ventricular beat/ventricular tachycardia (VT): when a beat originates in a ventricular focus, the activation wavefront spreads centrifugally from this site with a cell-to-cell propagation outside the specialized conduction tissue, producing a wide QRS complex (**Figs. 1** and **2**). As an exception, ectopic beats originating close to or in the bundle branches or Purkinje network show a narrower QRS complex, because a considerable part of the ventricular activation proceeds faster, over the specialized conduction tissue.
- Intraventricular conduction delay: conduction delay or block in one of the bundle branches or fascicles results in delayed activation of some regions of the ventricle, producing prolongation of the QRS complex; conduction delay is usually secondary to an anatomic/functional bundle branch block (**Fig. 3**). Rarely, it is an effect of drugs (most typically sodium channel blockers, such as class Ic antiarrhythmics or tricyclic antidepressants; **Fig. 4**) or electrolyte disturbances (eg, hyperkaliemia **Fig. 5**).
- Pacing: when a ventricular site (usually the right ventricle) is artificially paced, the depolarization wavefront proceeds centrifugally and slowly from the pacing site to the remaining ventricular myocardium (**Fig. 6**), similar to what is observed in ectopic ventricular beat. Therefore, the result of pacing is a wide QRS complex preceded by the pacing artifact. A narrower paced QRS complex is observed when the paced beat fuses with the normally conducted beat, when the pacing electrode is close to the His bundle area, or when the ventricles are simultaneously paced by two remote sites, as in biventricular pacing during cardiac resynchronization therapy.
- Ventricular preexcitation: a portion of the ventricular myocardium is activated early over an atrioventricular (AV) accessory pathway and fuses with the normal AV node-His-Purkinje activation wavefront to activate the entire ventricular myocardium (**Fig. 7**). The resulting fusion QRS complex is more or less wide, depending on the balance of the two AV conduction systems: the earlier the activation over the accessory pathway the wider the QRS complex.

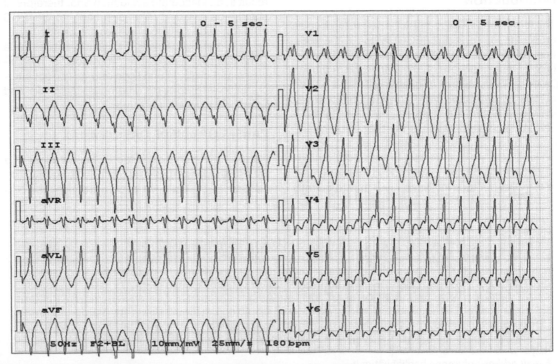

Fig. 1. Ventricular tachycardia with a right bundle branch pattern. Note the apparent "narrow" QRS complexes in the left precordial leads.

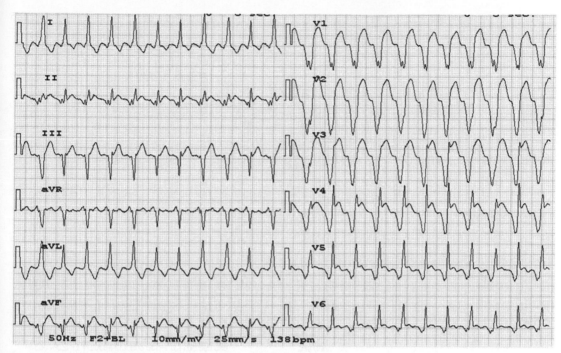

Fig. 2. Ventricular tachycardia with a left bundle branch block pattern.

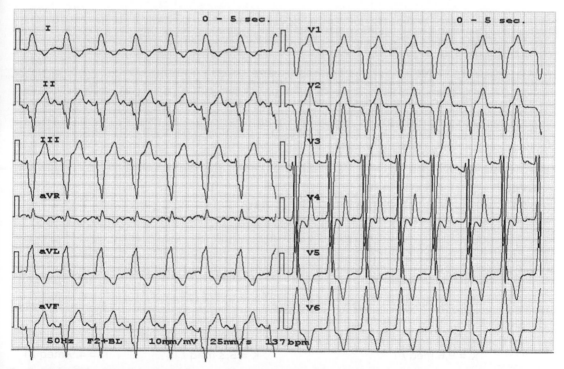

Fig. 3. Wide QRS complexes caused by intraventricular conduction delay (*left bundle branch block*).

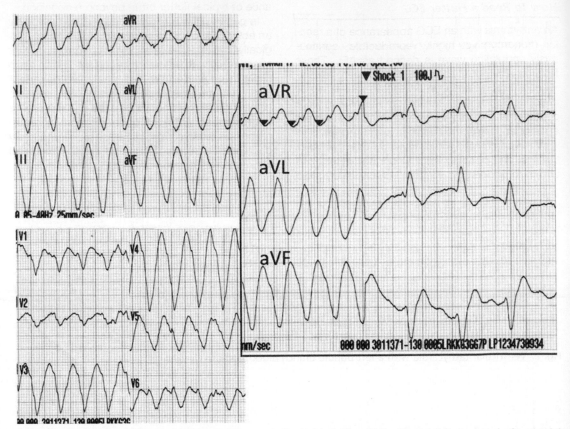

Fig. 4. Wide QRS complex tachycardia in a patient on flecainide before (*left*: 1:1 atrial flutter) and after (*right*) electrical cardioversion. Note in the right panel the very wide morphology of the QRS complex (qR in lead aVR).

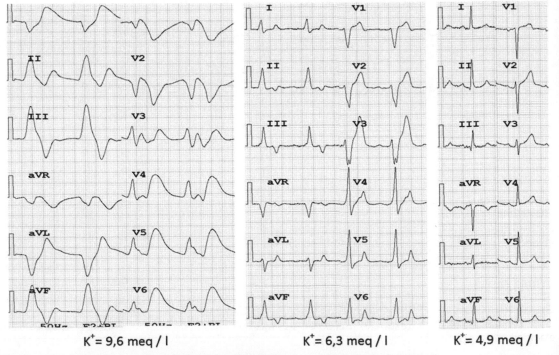

K⁺= 9,6 meq / l   K⁺= 6,3 meq / l   K⁺= 4,9 meq / l

Fig. 5. Wide QRS complexes caused by severe hyperkaliemia. See text for further details.

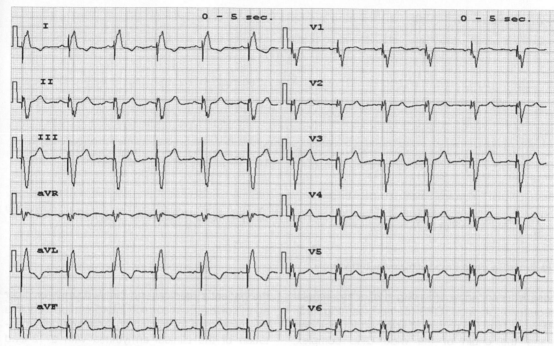

Fig. 6. Paced QRS complexes.

When interpreting an ECG with wide QRS complexes, it is important to consider the hypothesis of artifacts that simulate wide QRS complexes; in some cases, artifacts may show a regular and reproducible pattern, which makes the correct diagnosis even more difficult (**Fig. 8**).

ELECTROCARDIOGRAPHIC APPROACH TO A WIDE QRS COMPLEX

Wide QRS complexes can appear as premature beats (**Fig. 9**), late escape beats following a long pause (**Fig. 10**), couplets (**Fig. 11**), short runs of

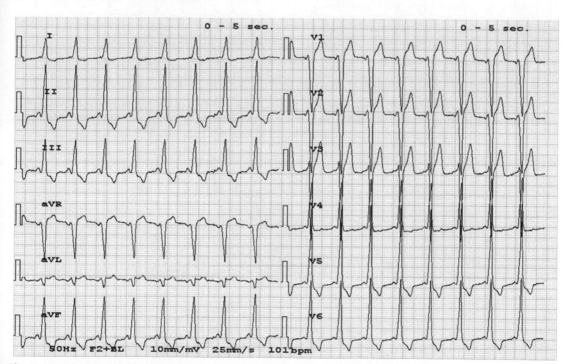

Fig. 7. Ventricular preexcitation over a right antero-septal accessory pathway.

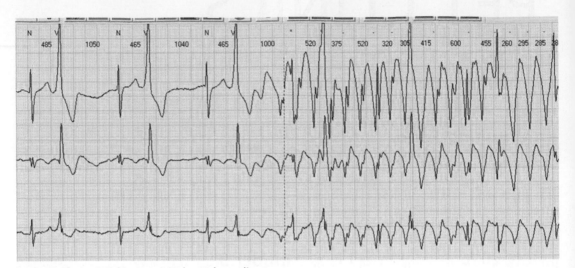

Fig. 8. Artifact mimicking ventricular tachycardia.

nonsustained tachycardia (**Fig. 12**), or as a regular sequence of wide QRS complexes (**Fig. 13**). Regardless of the pattern, it is important to understand the origin of the wide QRS complex, because the prognosis and treatment are different. As a general rule, when a wide QRS complex is present, a ventricular origin should always be suspected. There are some clinical elements that can help orient the diagnosis, such as the presence of a structural heart disease,

the patient's medical and family history, or older age; however, a correct interpretation requires adequate time for tracing analysis and documentation of the clinical arrhythmia with a 12-lead ECG is of utmost importance. Even if the patient is hemodynamically unstable, it would be important, if possible, to record a 12-lead ECG before restoring a hemodynamically stable rhythm to allow correct ECG interpretation, diagnosis, and subsequent therapy.

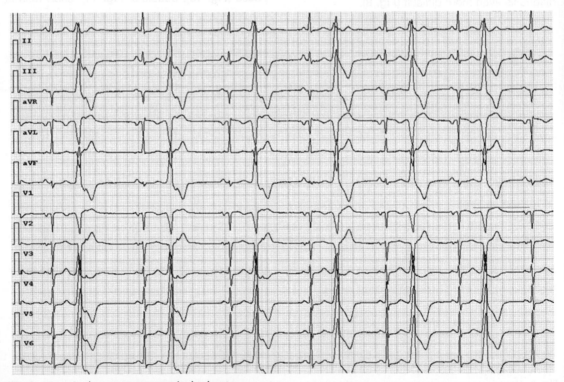

Fig. 9. Bigeminal premature ventricular beats.

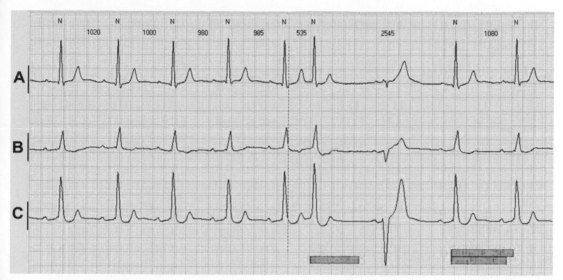

Fig. 10. Escape ventricular beat following a postextrasystolic compensatory pause.

When analyzing an ECG with a wide QRS complex, a systematic approach should be used, which includes the following steps (**Fig. 14**): (1) identification of each QRS present, their regularity, and their global representation in the 12 leads; (2) identification of atrial activity; (3) determination of the relationship between atrial and ventricular activity; and (4) in-depth evaluation of the wide QRS complex morphology (particularly in lead V₁ and in lead aVR). This approach allows reconstruction of the cardiac activation sequence, so that the timing of the sequential activation of the atria and ventricles is understood. This allows one to discriminate, for example, between atrial bigeminism with an ectopic P wave preceding a wide QRS complex caused by right bundle branch block (**Fig. 15**) and ventricular bigeminism with retrograde atrial activation, when the P wave

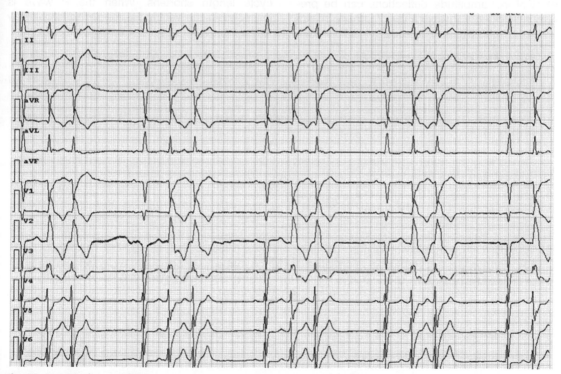

Fig. 11. Ventricular couplets.

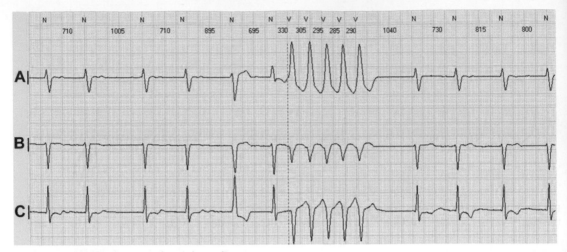

Fig. 12. Nonsustained ventricular tachycardia.

(negative in D$_2$) follows the wide QRS complex (**Fig. 16**). This is crucial also in the differential diagnosis of a WCT, to discriminate between VT and supraventricular tachycardia conducted with aberrancy, as explained in the following sections.

IDENTIFICATION OF ATRIAL ACTIVITY

The presence of wide QRS complexes complicates the identification of atrial activity. Peculiar alterations of the QRS complex with initial or terminal low-amplitude deflections can be present, mimicking a P wave (**Fig. 17**, *arrows* in lead

II and V$_6$). Moreover, the repolarization of a wide QRS complex is altered, making identification of a P wave even more difficult. It is important to carefully analyze each of the 12 leads, but lead II (**Fig. 18**) and V$_1$ (**Fig. 19**) are particularly helpful to identify atrial activity, especially when the P wave lies between the QRS complexes, during ventricular repolarization, or later during the isoelectric line. In the latter case, P wave identification is particularly easy, but, unfortunately, the duration of the isoelectric line decreases as the tachycardia cycle length shortens. When the P wave is inscribed in the ventricular repolarization, it may

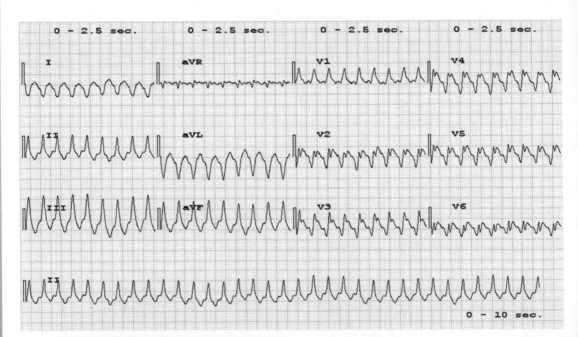

Fig. 13. Ventricular tachycardia.

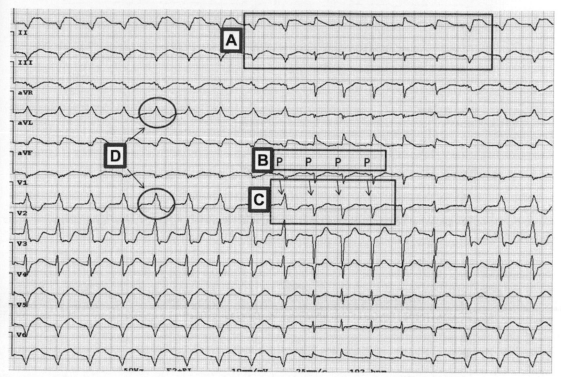

Fig. 14. Diagnostic steps to approach wide complex tachycardias. See text for complete details.

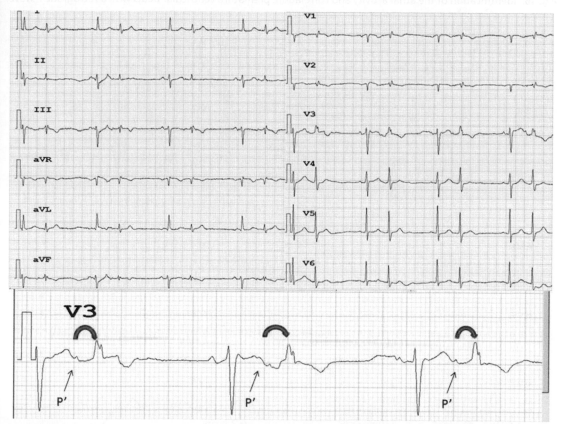

Fig. 15. Identification of atrial activity and correlation: premature atrial beats conducted with right bundle branch block.

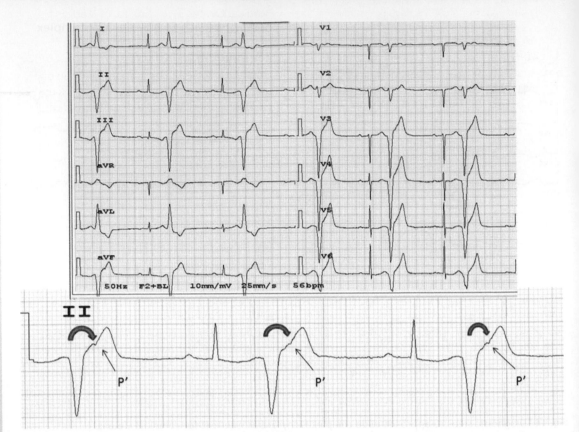

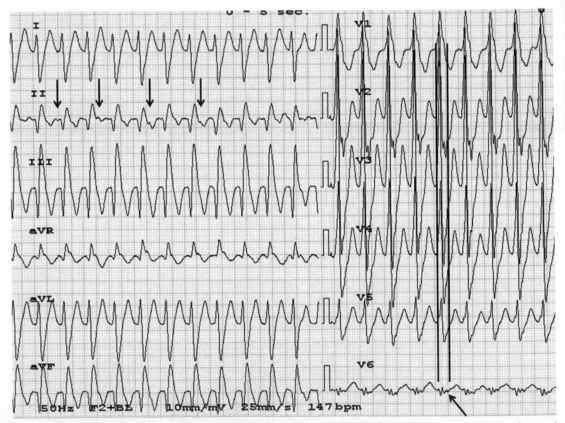

Fig. 16. Identification of the atrial activity and correlation: premature ventricular beats with a retrograde P wave.

Fig. 17. Ventricular tachycardia with dissociated atrial activity well evident in lead II. Note low-amplitude terminal deflections of the QRS in V_6, mimicking a P wave.

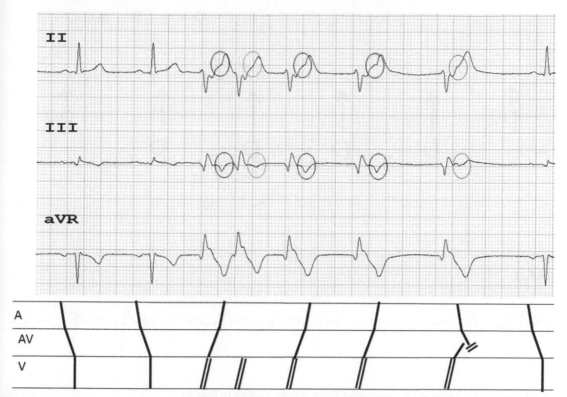

Fig. 18. Automatic ventricular rhythm. Retroconducted P waves inscribed during ventricular repolarization (*red circles*). Sinus P wave dissociated from the previous ventricular QRS (*blue circles*). Green circles represent the ascending T wave without any atrial activity inside.

appear as a fast "notch" that alters the ST segment or the T wave (see **Fig. 18**). When, despite all efforts, the P wave cannot be identified on the surface ECG, a bipolar esophageal recording of the atrial activity is helpful (**Fig. 20**). Alternatively, if the patient is in sinus rhythm, a dissociated jugular venous pulse can be the clinical equivalent of a dissociated atrial activity during a wide QRS complex tachycardia.

RELATIONSHIP BETWEEN ATRIAL AND VENTRICULAR ACTIVITY

When the atrial activity is identified, it is important determine the relationship between the atrial and the ventricular activity, which is the cornerstone of the interpretation of an ECG with wide QRS complexes. Indeed, when ventriculoatrial (VA) dissociation is present (atrial activity slower and independent of ventricular activity), the diagnosis of a ventricular origin is made (see **Figs. 20** and **21**). Moreover, the presence of a second-degree VA block (QRS complexes greater than retrogradely conducted P waves) suggests a ventricular origin of the tachycardia (**Fig. 22**). Conversely, it is not possible to establish the origin of the tachycardia in case of a 1:1 relationship between the atrial

and ventricular activity. In approximately 50% of cases, there is a stable 1:1 relationship between the atrial and ventricular activity during VT. Vagal maneuvers and adenosine may help by blocking AV node conduction (**Fig. 23**). More specifically, if they produce VA dissociation or a second-degree VA block appears, the rhythm has a ventricular origin. Conversely, if they result in a second- or third-degree AV block (P waves more frequent than QRS complexes), this proves the supraventricular origin of the tachycardia. Similarly, termination of a wide QRS complex tachycardia by vagal stimulation supports the hypothesis that the arrhythmia is sustained by a supraventricular reentry tachycardia involving the AV node (**Fig. 24**). Finally, when the onset of a wide QRS complex tachycardia has been recorded, identifying and understanding the sequence of the atrial and ventricular activation is key to clarify the arrhythmia mechanism (**Fig. 25**).

MORPHOLOGIC CHANGES OF THE WIDE QRS COMPLEX: CAPTURE AND FUSION BEATS

If the atrial activity is not easily identifiable and the relationship between the atrial and ventricular activity is unclear, the next step is looking for

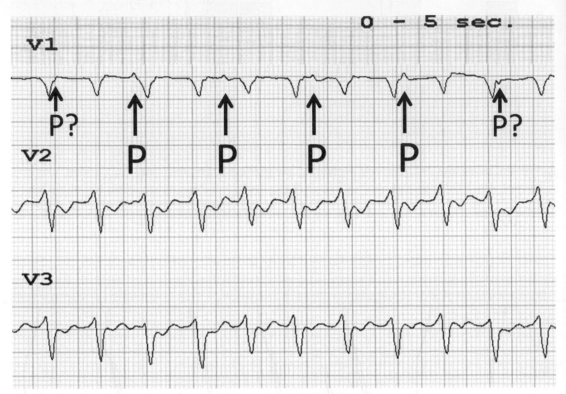

Fig. 19. Ventricular tachycardia. Dissociated atrial activity evident in lead V₁.

morphologic changes of the wide QRS complex. The most important clue is given by narrowing or even normalization of the QRS complex observed in a single or consecutive beats. To do so, it is important to obtain a prolonged ECG recording, possibly with a vertical display of the 12 leads, which may increase the chance to detect this phenomenon (see **Fig. 25**). These changes are caused by partial (fusion) or complete (capture) depolarization of the ventricular myocardium by a supraventricular beat (usually a sinus beat), which remains dissociated during VT and is conducted anterograde over the normal AV conduction system. When capture or fusion beats are observed, a P wave can usually be detected before the narrower QRS complex (see **Figs. 14; Fig. 26**). This phenomenon can only occur in the presence of VA dissociation, which is pathognomonic of a ventricular origin of the wide QRS complex tachycardia. Capture and fusion beats are identified more easily in slower wide QRS complex tachycardias: the longer the tachycardia cycle length, the wider the excitable gap between two subsequent ventricular depolarizations, the easier for a supraventricular beat conducted over the normal AV conduction system to narrow or normalize the subsequent beat during VT. Indeed, fusion and capture beats are more frequently observed in the presence of slower idioventricular rhythms than during a fast VT.

MORPHOLOGIC CHANGES OF THE QRS COMPLEX ACCORDING TO THE CYCLE LENGTH: ASHMAN PHENOMENON

A wide QRS complex occasionally can originate from a supraventricular beat that is conducted with a functional bundle branch block. This is the Ashman phenomenon, which states that aberrancy is more easily achieved after a long/short sequence of the RR intervals. The long/short cycle sequences are particularly frequent during atrial fibrillation, where the Ashman phenomenon is fundamental for the diagnosis of aberrancy of intraventricular conduction (**Fig. 27**).[1] In this case, aberrant conduction occurs predictably and the following elements are necessary: first, a particularly long R-R cycle preceding a QRS complex, so that the effective refractory period of one of two bundle branches is prolonged (see **Fig. 27**, *left*); second, a particularly short coupling interval between the wide QRS complex and the last narrow QRS beat, so that one of two branches is still refractory (see **Fig. 27**, *right*).

The longer the preceding cycle and the shorter coupling interval, the higher the probability of

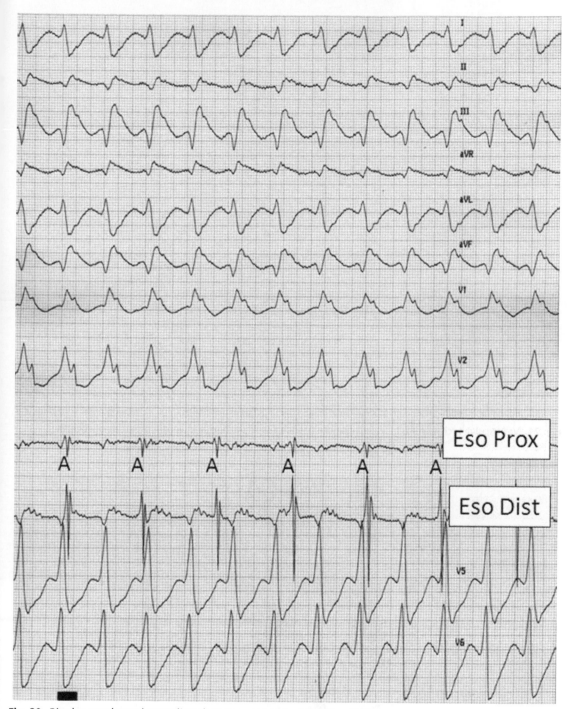

Fig. 20. Bipolar esophageal recording showing ventriculoatrial dissociation.

aberrant conduction. Once aberrant conduction has occurred in the first beat after a short coupling interval for the Ashman phenomenon, it can persist even for cycle lengths longer than the effective refractory period of the blocked bundle branch. This occurs because of continuous retrograde concealed conduction into the anterogradely blocked bundle branch, which, therefore, is refractory to the next oncoming supraventricular impulse (linking phenomenon; **Fig. 28**). If not properly recognized, the occurrence of linking is misleading and a

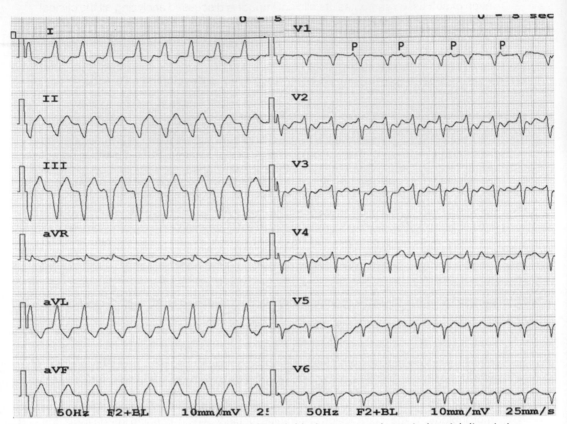

Fig. 21. Ventricular tachycardia. In V$_1$ left bundle branch block pattern and ventriculoatrial dissociation.

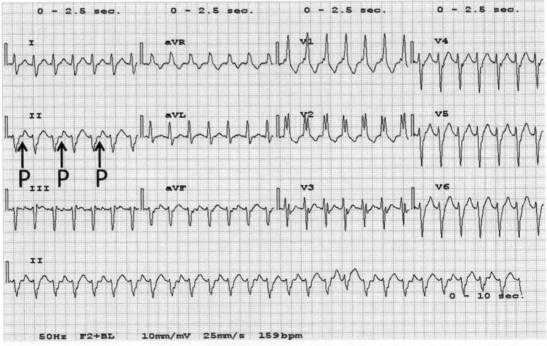

Fig. 22. Fascicular ventricular tachycardia. QRS with right bundle branch block in V$_1$ and left axial deviation. 2:1 ventriculoatrial block is present (*arrows*: retrograde P wave).

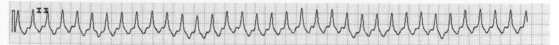

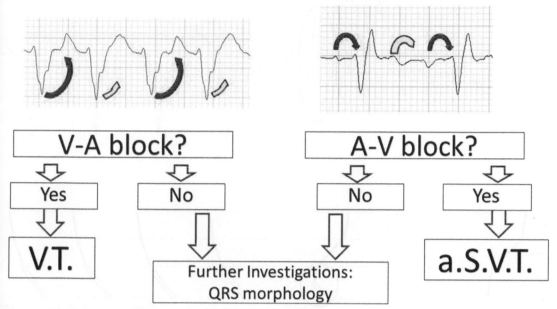

Wide QRS: AtrioVentricular Relationship
(Spontaneous, Vagal Tone or Adenosine)

V-A block?

Yes → No →

V.T.

A-V block?

No → Yes →

Further Investigations:
QRS morphology

a.S.V.T.

Fig. 23. Effect of vagal maneuvers or adenosine in wide QRS complex tachycardia. See text for further details. aSVT, aberrant supraventricular tachycardia; A-V, atrioventricular; V-A, ventriculoatrial; V.T., ventricular tachycardia.

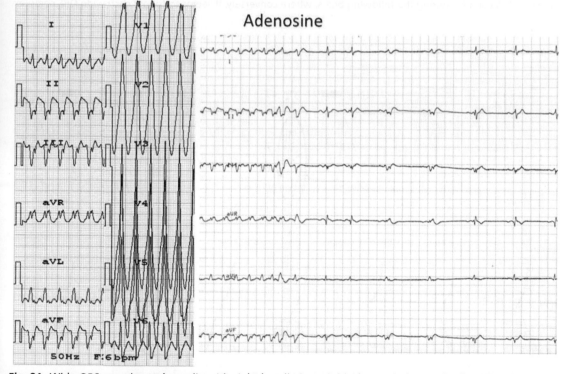

Adenosine

Fig. 24. Wide QRS complex tachycardia with right bundle branch block morphology in lead V₁. Termination of the tachycardia with adenosine, suggests an antidromic atrioventricular tachycardia (pre-excitation is evident upon sinus rhythm regression).

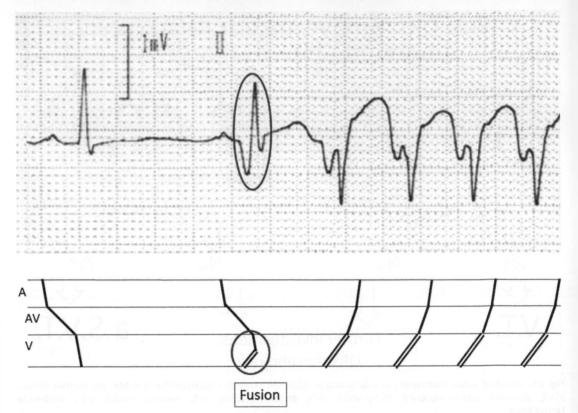

Fig. 25. Initiation of a wide QRS complex tachycardia with a fusion beat (*red circles*); there is no P wave preceding the wide QRS complex during the following beats, where conversely, it seems to follow each wide QRS complex.

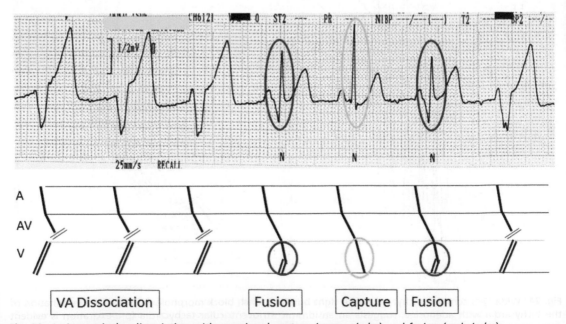

Fig. 26. Atrioventricular dissociation with occasional capture (*green circles*) and fusion (*red circles*).

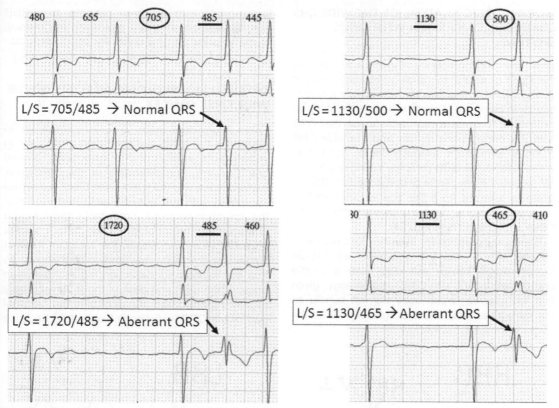

Fig. 27. Ashman phenomenon (long/short cycle) during atrial fibrillation. (*Left*) The role of the long cycle. (*Right*) The role of the short cycle. See text for complete details.

supraventricular arrhythmia can be misdiagnosed as ventricular. Aberrant conduction may terminate for further prolongation of the cycle length of the tachycardia or for the occurrence of the "reverse"

Ashman phenomenon (short/long sequence), characterized by a short cycle followed by long cycle, with subsequent normalization of the QRS complex (see **Fig. 28**).

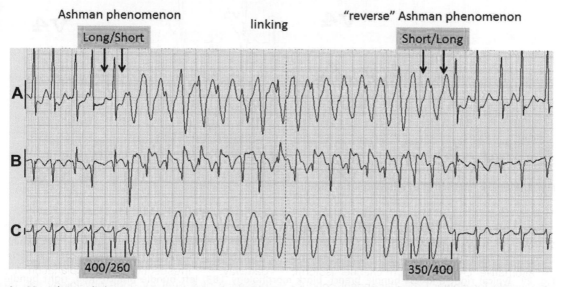

Fig. 28. Ashman, linking and reverse Ashman phenomena during atrial fibrillation. See text for details.

MORPHOLOGIC ANALYSIS OF THE WIDE QRS COMPLEX: COMPARISON WITH SINUS RHYTHM

When the QRS complex during sinus rhythm has the same or similar morphology of that observed during the WCT, this arrhythmia is likely supraventricular in origin (see **Fig. 4**). When ventricular preexcitation is present, comparison of the QRS complex during sinus rhythm and the wide QRS complex arrhythmia, although useful, has limitations. Indeed, the QRS complex during antidromic AV reentrant tachycardia or preexcited atrial fibrillation is different from the one in sinus rhythm because of a higher degree of preexcitation during these arrhythmias (see **Fig. 24**).

There are exceptions to this rule. For example, a patient with a baseline complete left bundle branch block (LBBB) can also have a bundle branch reentry VT with LBBB morphology, given that tachycardia circuit uses the left bundle as the retrograde limb and the right bundle as the anterograde limb. In these patients, the LBBB (usually associated with a prolonged PR interval) is the expression of a distal AV conduction disease, which facilities the aforementioned reentry.

DETAILED MORPHOLOGIC ANALYSIS OF THE WIDE QRS COMPLEX

When analyzing a wide QRS, it is important to determine if it looks like aberration or not. When widening of the QRS complex is caused by bundle branch block, depolarization of the ventricular mass ipsilateral to the conduction block is delayed compared with the normally activated ventricle: the activation pattern is predictable, generating a characteristic morphology of the QRS complex (**Fig. 29**). More specifically, the vector of the first ventricular activation may remain unchanged, so that the intrinsicoid deflection (interval between onset of the QRS and peak of the R wave) is only slightly modified; on the contrary, the terminal part of the QRS is distinctly fragmented because

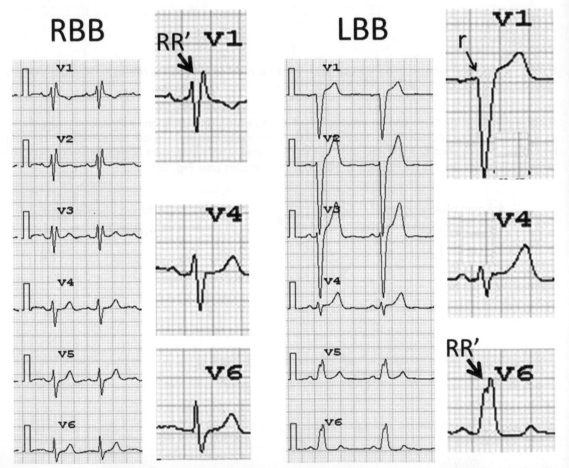

Fig. 29. Typical right and left bundle branch block morphology. LBB, left bundle branch; RBB, right bundle branch.

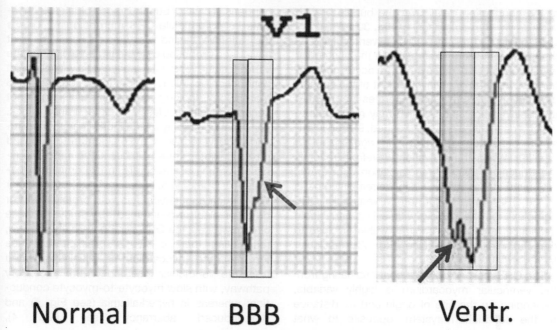

Fig. 30. Intrinsicoid deflection in a normal QRS (*left*), wide QRS caused by conduction delay (*middle*), and wide QRS during ventricular tachycardia (*right*). See text for complete details. BBB, bundle branch block.

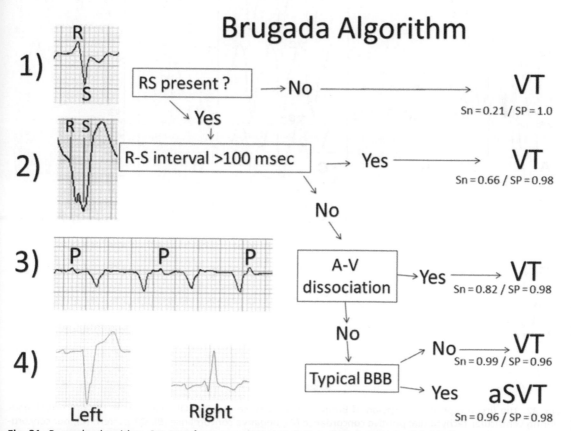

Fig. 31. Brugada algorithm. See text for a complete description. BBB, bundle branch block.

of the conduction delay over the bundle branch (*blue arrow* in *middle* panel of **Fig. 30**). When the QRS complex originates from a ventricular site, the initial activation takes place in the ventricular myocardium, with myocyte-to-myocyte conduction and minimal or no involvement of the specific conduction system. This generates fragmented and delayed activation, which may result in low-voltage deflections and a prolonged, slurred intrinsicoid deflection (*red arrow* in *right* panel of **Fig. 30**). When the activation wavefront reaches the Purkinje network, depolarization accelerates with faster deflection waves in the remaining parts of the QRS complex. Of note, a ventricular QRS complex may be narrow with a fast intrinsicoid deflection in case the origin is within or close to the Purkinje network (see **Fig. 22** fascicular tachycardia).

The QRS morphology of a beat originating from the ventricular myocardium is highly variable, depending on the site of origin and its distance to the conduction system, opposite to what

happens in case of bundle branch block, which results in reproducible QRS morphologies. This is the rationale behind the various algorithms that have been proposed over the years to differentiate VT from supraventricular tachycardia with aberrant conduction in WCT, which focus on the QRS morphology, looking for specific ECG signs not consistent with a classic bundle branch block. The most commonly used algorithms are the Brugada and Vereckei (or aVR) algorithm (discussed next). Of note, none of these QRS morphology-based criteria are accurate in discriminating between VT and rare forms of supraventricular WCT, such as tachycardias with preexcitation or drug- or electrolyte-induced aberrancy. In these circumstances, the QRS can be wide and bizarre, resembling that of VT: in preexcitation (see **Fig. 24**), the myocardium is initially activated from the ventricular insertion of the accessory pathway, with slow myocyte-to-myocyte conduction; whereas in hyperkaliemia (see **Fig. 5**) and drug-induced aberrancy (see **Fig. 4**),

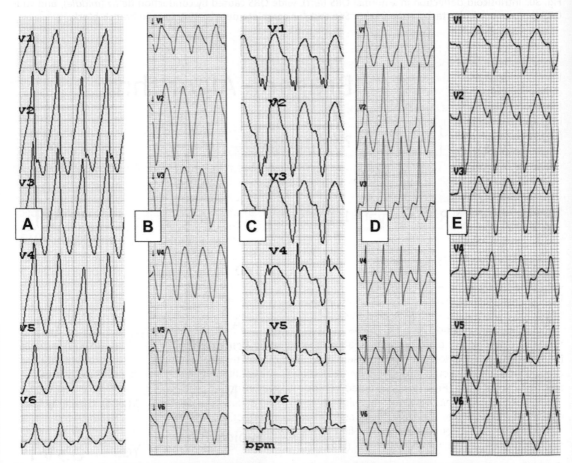

Fig. 32. The first morphologic criterion of Brugada: concordance. Possible QRS patterns in the precordial leads during ventricular tachycardia: positive concordance (*A*), negative concordance (*B*), QR pattern (*C*), nonconcordance (*D*, *E*).

interventricular conduction delay is profound and does not follow a predictable pattern, persisting throughout the QRS complex.

BRUGADA ALGORITHM

The Brugada algorithm takes into account the morphology of the QRS complex in the precordial leads and the presence of VA dissociation.[2] There are three morphologic criteria that point to the diagnosis of VT (**Fig. 31**) as discussed next.

The first criterion is absence of a RS complex in all precordial leads (concordance). During VT, there are three possible patterns throughout the chest leads (**Fig. 32**): (1) positive concordance (only R waves; see **Fig. 32**A), (2) negative concordance (only QS waves; see **Fig. 32**B), and (3) a QR morphology pattern (a variant of the negative concordance pattern, typically associated with an old myocardial infarction; see **Fig. 32**C).

There are some exceptions to the rule that a concordant pattern defines a ventricular origin. More specifically, a positive concordance is present in antidromic AV reentry tachycardia sustained by a posterior accessory pathway; and a negative concordance can be seen during apical stimulation and, therefore, be present in pacemaker-mediated tachycardias.

The absence of an RS complex in all precordial leads (first morphologic criterion of Brugada) has a high specificity (100%), but low sensitivity (21%), and when it is not verified, the origin of tachycardia remains uncertain (see **Fig. 32**D, E).

The second criterion is intrinsicoid deflection greater than 100 milliseconds in at least one of the precordial leads. This criterion is based on the original observation by Kindwall and colleagues[3] who found that in LBBB morphology WCT, an intrinsicoid deflection in V_1 greater than 60 milliseconds, was specific for VT. Brugada extended this concept to all the precordial leads and to every QRS complex morphology and determined that a cutoff value of 100 milliseconds discriminated VT from supraventricular tachycardia with a specificity of 98% and a sensitivity of 66% (**Fig. 33**).

The third criterion is morphology criteria for VT present in both the right and left precordial leads. In right bundle branch block morphology WCT

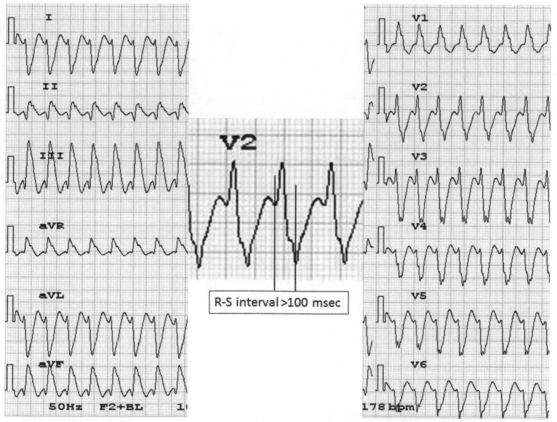

Fig. 33. The second morphologic criterion of Brugada. Prolonged intrinsicoid deflection in precordial leads (R-S >100 ms) suggestive of ventricular tachycardia.

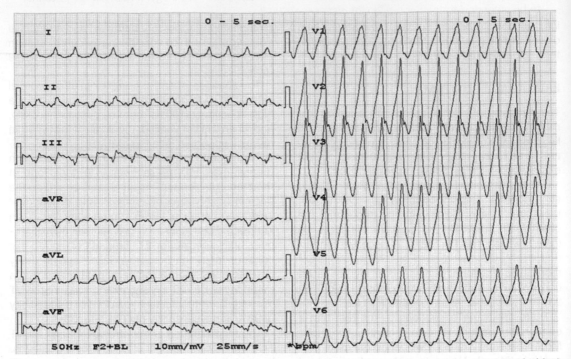

Fig. 34. The third morphologic criterion of Brugada. Ventricular tachycardia right bundle branch block morphology: monophasic R in V$_1$.

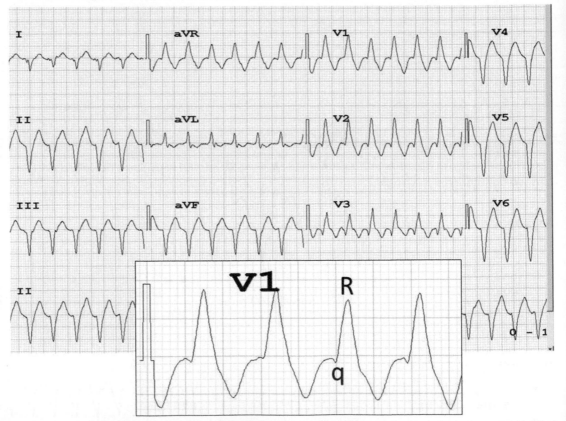

Fig. 35. The third morphologic criterion of Brugada. Ventricular tachycardia with right bundle branch block morphology: wide QRS complex with qR in V$_1$ and rS in V$_6$.

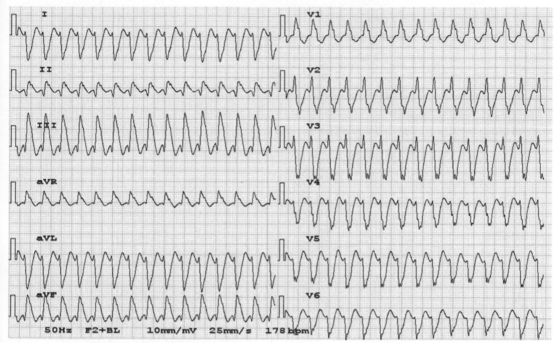

Fig. 36. The third morphologic criterion of Brugada. Ventricular tachycardia with right bundle branch block morphology: Rr′ in V₁ and QS complex in V₆.

(QRS mostly positive in V_1), VT is favored in the presence of (1) a monophasic R (**Fig. 34**), or biphasic qR (**Fig. 35**) or Rs complex in V_1; (2) an RSR′ pattern in V_1 with the R peak being higher in amplitude than the R′ peak (**Fig. 36**); and (3) a rS complex in lead V_6 (see **Fig. 21**). In LBBB morphology WCT (QRS mostly negative in V_1), VT is more likely in the presence of a wide R wave (>30 ms) in lead V_1 or V_2 (**Fig. 37**), a slurred or notched downstroke of the S wave in V_1 or V_2, intrinsicoid deflection lower than 60 milliseconds in V_1 or V_2, and a Q wave (QS or QR complexes) in V_6 (**Fig. 38**).

In the Brugada algorithm, a further step is the ECG demonstration of VA dissociation, which is usually applied between the second and third morphologic criterion (see **Fig. 31**).

VERECKEI ALGORITHM

The algorithm proposed by Vereckei and co-workers[4] adopts the conventional criteria of VA dissociation together with the morphologic analysis of the QRS complex in aVR. Of note, aVR is the unipolar lead from the right arm, which shows a predominantly negative QRS complex during

normal sinus rhythm. The morphologic criteria in aVR are as follows (**Fig. 39**):

- Criterion 1: presence of a dominant initial R wave (an R wave that represents the largest deflection of the QRS complex); this finding proves a substantial deviation of the ventricular activation sequence, consistent with a rhythm originating in the ventricular myocardium
- Criterion 2: presence of an initial nondominant Q or R wave with a duration greater than 40 milliseconds; this finding suggests the occurrence of slow conduction at the beginning of ventricular depolarization, which is typically observed in a rhythm of ventricular origin.
- Criterion 3: presence of a notch on the initial downstroke in a predominantly negative QRS complex (QS or QR); similar to the previous criterion, this finding is an expression of the delay in the initial ventricular activation that occurs during VT.
- Criterion 4: total amplitude[a] of the QRS in the first 40 milliseconds (V_i) less than the total amplitude of the QRS in last 40 milliseconds (V_t) of the QRS, or V_i/V_t <1; with aberration, the initial ventricular activation is mediated

[a]Vi and Vt are calculated as the sum of all the QRS deflections, regardless if they are positive or negative.

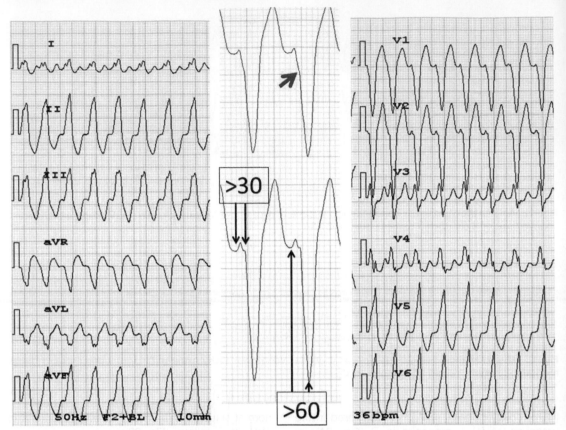

Fig. 37. The third morphologic criterion of Brugada. Ventricular tachycardia with left bundle branch block morphology: initial R wave longer than 30 ms and R-S longer than 60 ms. The red arrow indicates a notched down stroke of the S wave.

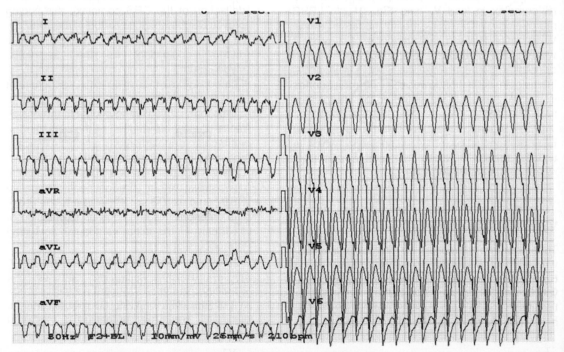

Fig. 38. Ventricular tachycardia with left bundle branch block morphology.

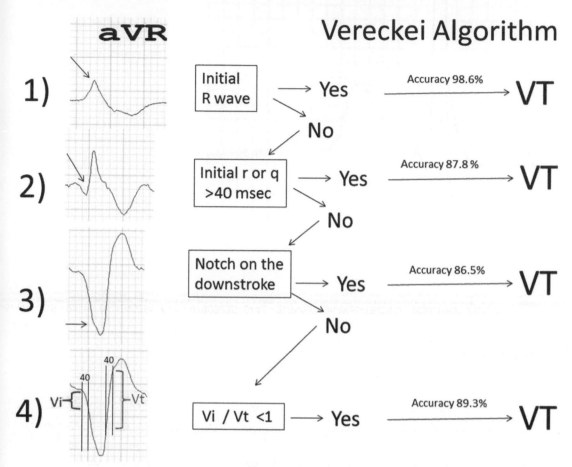

Fig. 39. Vereckei algorithm. See text for a complete description. Vi, total amplitude of the QRS in the first 40 ms; Vt, total amplitude of the QRS in last 40 ms.

by the His-Purkinje system, producing an initial depolarization wavefront much greater than the terminal one

SUMMARY

When a wide QRS complex is observed, a ventricular origin should be always suspected. Some clinical elements, such as the presence of structural heart disease, patient's and family history, or age, may in some way help orient the diagnosis, which, however, has to be made based merely on ECG criteria. A correct interpretation requires adequate time for tracing analysis, and adequate documentation of the arrhythmia. Therefore, if the patient is hemodynamically unstable, an optimal strategy is to record as much as possible of the spontaneous arrhythmia on a 12-lead ECG and then, after restoring a hemodynamically stable rhythm, start or continue with a thorough tracing interpretation.

REFERENCES

1. Gouaux JL, Ashman R. Auricular fibrillation with aberration simulating ventricular paroxysmal tachycardia. Am Heart J 1947;34(3):366–73.

2. Brugada P, Brugada J, Mont L, et al. A new approach to the differential diagnosis of a regular tachycardia with a wide QRS complex. Circulation 1991;83(5):1649–59.

3. Kindwall KE, Brown J, Josephson ME. Electrocardiographic criteria for ventricular tachycardia in wide complex left bundle branch block morphology tachycardias. Am J Cardiol 1988;61(15):1279–83.

4. Vereckei A, Duray G, Szénási G, et al. New algorithm using only lead aVR for differential diagnosis of wide QRS complex tachycardia. Heart Rhythm 2008;5(1):89–98.

Fig. 39. Vereckei algorithm. See text for a complete description. Vi, total amplitude of the first 40 ms; Vt, total amplitude of the QRS in last 40 ms.

Normal Ventricular Repolarization and QT Interval
Ionic Background, Modifiers, and Measurements

Emanuela T. Locati, MD, PhD[a],*, Giuseppe Bagliani, MD[b,c],
Luigi Padeletti, MD[d,e]

KEYWORDS

- Ventricular repolarization • QT interval • J point • ST segment • T wave • U wave • Electric memory
- T wave alternans

KEY POINTS

- Ventricular repolarization is a cellular electrophysiological process expressed in the electrocardiogram as the QT interval.
- Intramural differences in the ventricular repolarization are at the base of ST and T waves in the electrocardiogram.
- The QT interval is variable, and many factors affect its duration: heart rate, autonomic nervous activity, age, and gender are the main determinants.
- Many criteria correct the duration of QT interval for heart rate.
- Conditions provoking repolarization abnormalities (QT prolongation) are ionic changes, drugs, cardiac/noncardiac diseases, and genetic background (long QT syndromes).

INTRODUCTION: SIGNIFICANCE AND ROLE OF VENTRICULAR REPOLARIZATION

The QT interval on the surface electrocardiogram (ECG) represents the sum of depolarization and repolarization processes of the ventricles. Although the ventricular activation, reflected by the QRS complex on the surface ECG, corresponds to the fast spreading of the depolarization through the ventricular muscle, the ventricular repolarization, reflected by the ST segment and T wave, represents the recovery period of the ventricles, when they recruit the electrical forces activated during the depolarization while the ventricles are protected against a reexcitation happening before the mechanical function is completed.[1,2] Although ventricular depolarization is mainly based on very fast inward sodium-dependent currents, ventricular repolarization mainly depends on the transmembrane outward transport of potassium ions to reestablish the endocellular electronegativity (**Fig. 1**). Outward potassium channels represent a heterogeneous family of ionic carriers, whose global kinetics is modulated by heart rate and

[a] Electrophysiology Unit, Cardiology Division, Cardiovascular Department, ASST GOM Niguarda Hospital, Piazza Ospedale Maggiore, 3, 20162 Milano, Italy; [b] Arrhythmology Unit, Cardiology Department, Foligno General Hospital, Via Massimo Arcamone, 06034 Foligno (PG), Italy; [c] Cardiovascular Diseases Department, University of Perugia, Piazza Menghini 1, 06129 Perugia Italy; [d] Heart and Vessels Department, University of Florence, Largo Brambilla, 3, 50134 Florence, Italy; [e] IRCCS Multimedica, Cardiology Department, Via Milanese, 300, 20099 Sesto San Giovanni, Italy
* Corresponding author.
E-mail address: emanuelateresa.locati@ospedaleniguarda.it

Card Electrophysiol Clin 9 (2017) 487–513
http://dx.doi.org/10.1016/j.ccep.2017.05.007
1877-9182/17/© 2017 Elsevier Inc. All rights reserved.

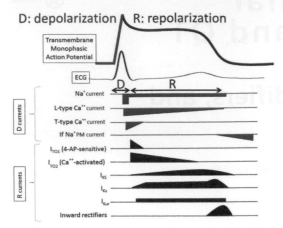

Fig. 1. Cardiac ionic currents and respective ion channels clones responsible for the generation of the action potential. Inward currents (positive charges moving into the cells) are displayed as downward and drawn in red, outward currents (positive charges moving out of the cells) as upward in blue (the amplitudes are not in scale).

sympathetic nervous activity, and affected by several cardiac and noncardiac drugs and disease conditions, and by gene mutations determining distinct channellopathies.[3–5]

Even in normal conditions, *ventricular repolarization is more heterogeneous than ventricular depolarization*. The presence of progressive shorter repolarization in areas of later activation tends to *synchronize ventricular repolarization*, and it may be an important physiologic mechanism in the prevention of arrhythmias. Perturbations of ventricular depolarization and repolarization (due to ischemia, bundle branch block, preexcitation, extrasystolic beats, drugs, or genetic abnormalities of cardiac ion channels) can alter the J and particularly T wave configuration and prolong QT interval duration, favoring the arrhythmogenesis.[6,7]

There has been great interest in prolongation of ventricular repolarization in relation to the genesis of life-threatening ventricular arrhythmias, both in acquired and in congenital conditions, characterized by prolonged QT interval, abnormal T-wave configuration, and increased dispersion of QT interval duration, generally defined as "long QT syndromes" (LQTS).[7–10]

In more recent years, there has been major focus on abnormalities of the early phase of ventricular repolarization, defined as "J-wave syndromes," among which the best known is the "Brugada syndrome" (BrS).[10–12]

The most recently recognized disorder of ventricular repolarization associated with ventricular tachyarrhythmias, syncope, and sudden death is the "short QT syndrome" (SQTS), a rare genetically

inherited cardiac channelopathy on the same spectrum as other familial arrhythmogenic diseases.[13]

ELECTROPHYSIOLOGICAL BASIS OF NORMAL VENTRICULAR REPOLARIZATION

The QT interval, measured from the onset of the Q wave to the end of the T wave, reflects the total duration of the ventricular electrical systole. The QT interval includes the ventricular *depolarization time* (reflected by the QRS duration), and the *repolarization time* (reflected by the JT interval and the T wave). Several attempts have been made to correlate the QT interval waveforms recorded on surface ECG with the action potentials originating from different cardiac sites.[1–3,14,15]

Ionic Currents Determining the Cardiac Action Potential

The most distinctive feature of cardiac action potential is the *plateau phase*. The *plateau* is crucial to determine the strength and duration of myocardium contraction, to set the proper relationship between systolic contraction and diastolic filling times, and to provide a *cardio-protective window* in which reexcitation cannot occur. Ventricular action potentials have, with respect to the atrium, a relatively stable and longer plateau phase and a domelike shape. The action potential shape varies in different parts of the ventricle and throughout the ventricular wall. Furthermore, the shape varies over time depending on heart rate, as a fast heart rate speeds up repolarization. The different cardiac ion channels play well-defined roles in shaping the action potential. During the normal cardiac cycle, *inward movement of positive ions* (mainly sodium and calcium currents) induces cell depolarization cells, whereas *outward flow of positive charges* (mainly potassium currents) induces repolarization (see **Fig. 1**). The stability of cardiac electrical activity, and mainly the plateau phase, is secured by some degree of redundancy in combination with the tight voltage-gated dependence regulation of ion channels. The various potassium channels involved in repolarization of the action potential represent a good example of such redundancy, and this phenomenon has been described as the *"repolarization reserve."*[3–5]

The cardiac action potential is divided into 5 distinct phases (phases 0–4), with different currents active in each phase.

Phase 0

The abrupt shift in membrane potential in a positive direction (depolarization) that initiates the systolic period, is driven by influx of Na^+ (I_{na}), through the NaV1.5 channel encoded by the gene SCN5A, generally insensitive to tetrodotoxin.

Phase 1

The transient early repolarization following the repolarization, most prominent in atria and the ventricular epicardium, is caused by inactivation of NaV1.5 channels in combination with activation of transient voltage-gated K currents (I_{to}) that can further be divided into $I_{to,fast}$ and $I_{to,slow}$. Functionally, the fast repolarization in phase 1 contributes to increasing the driving gradient for Ca^{+2} into the cardiac myocytes. Mainly in atria, an additional ultrarapid current called I_{Kur} contributes to early repolarization. I_{Kur} is conducted by KV1.5 potassium channels, and due to its slow inactivation, plays a role during phases 1 to 3, partly responsible for the triangular action potential shape of the atria compared with the ventricles.[3,4]

Phase 2

The long-lasting depolarized plateau of the cardiac action potential is a prerequisite for excitation-contraction coupling and is caused by a balance between outward K^+ currents and inward currents through voltage-gated Ca^{+2} channels. The latter are located in the t-tubules, and the Ca^{+2} influx through these channels activates ryanodine receptors located just below in the sarcoplasmic reticulum. The subsequent Ca^{+2}-dependent Ca^{+2} release from intracellular stores triggers muscle contraction. Phase 2 is terminated by a voltage-dependent and Ca^{+2}/calmodulin-dependent slow inactivation of CaV1.2 combined with the simultaneous activation of K^+ channels including I_{KR} and I_{KS}. To a lesser extent, the Ca^{+2} influx in the early part of phase 2 is also transported by the electrogenic Na^+/Ca^{+2} exchanger.[3,4]

Phase 3

Phase 3 represents the repolarization from plateau phase to resting membrane potential. The repolarization is caused by the balance between inactivating Ca^{+2} current and rising K^+ channels tilting quickly toward the latter. In humans and other large mammals, 3 different potassium currents called I_{Kr}, I_{Ks}, and I_{K1} are mainly responsible for repolarization. They have diverse but partly overlapping functions, and to stress the latter they have often been called the "repolarization reserve."[3,4] The partly overlapping function of these 3 currents driving phase 3 repolarization occurs on the basis of very different gating properties.

The voltage-gated current I_{Kr}, encoded by KCNH2 gene, and also called hERG, is characterized by a relatively fast activation on depolarization, then a rapid inactivation that renders the channel virtually nonconductive during phases 0 to 2 of the action potential, while the initial repolarization will release I_{Kr} from inactivation and reopen the channel, allowing I_{Kr} to conduct currents during both phase 3 and the early part of the diastolic phase 4 of the action potential.

I_{Ks}, encoded by the KCNQ1 gene, is also voltage-gated, opening at potentials positive to −20 mV and activating slowly, and in contrast to I_{Kr}, not inactivating during phase 3. These properties enable I_{Ks} to build up slowly during phase 2 and to become one of the key K^+ conductance in phase 3.

The third current, I_{K1}, encoded by the KCNJ2 gene, is only indirectly voltage sensitive and will contribute particularly to repolarization in the late part of phase 3. I_{k1} is an inward rectifying potassium current, which stabilizes the resting membrane potential and is responsible for shaping the final repolarization of the action potential. Several studies suggest I_{K1} plays a role in ventricular arrhythmias. I_{K1} stays open during diastole and is important for setting the resting membrane potential.

In addition to the "repolarization reserve currents," I_{Kr}, I_{Ks}, and I_{K1}, other potassium currents can have a significant impact on repolarization of cardiac action potentials, such as I_{Kur} and IK_{ACh}, and IK_{ATP}. Under normal physiologic conditions, the intracellular ATP level is sufficiently high to inhibit the channels, but during hypoxia and ischemia, the intracellular ATP level drops and may result in an activation of IK_{ATP}, resulting in triangulation of the action potential.[3,4]

Phase 4

Phase 4 is the interval between full repolarization and initiation of the next action potential. In this diastolic interval, the cardiac myocytes are at resting membrane potential, and the charge movements are primarily conducted via various K^+ channels, including 2-pore motif leak channels (I_{leak}). Additional K^+ channels with slow deactivation kinetics also remain open in the initial part of phase 4. These K^+ currents will counteract possible depolarizing events from delayed afterdepolarizations. However, the inhibitory force of the K^+ conductance is not enough to withstand massive depolarizing stimuli arising from a new wave of action potentials. Prolongation of the effective refractory period through K^+ channel inhibition together with Na^+ channel inactivation remains the more efficient mechanism against reentrant arrhythmias.[3,4]

Intramural Differences in the Action Potential Duration

It has long been recognized that endocardium has longer action potentials than epicardium.[1-3] More recently it has been demonstrated that ventricular myocardium is composed of 3 electrophysiologically and functionally distinct cell types:

- Epicardial
- Midmyocardial (M)
- Endocardial

These 3 principal ventricular myocardial cell types (**Fig. 2**)[3,15] differ with respect to phase 1 and phase 3 repolarization characteristics. Ventricular epicardial and M, but not endocardial, cells generally display a prominent phase 1, due to a large 4-aminopyridine–sensitive transient outward current (I_{to}), giving the action potential a spike and dome or notched configuration. Regional differences in I_{to} have now been directly demonstrated in many species, including human ventricular myocytes. Differences in the magnitude of action potential notch and corresponding differences in I_{to} have also been described between right and left ventricular epicardial and M cells. This distinction may explain why BrS, a channelopathy-mediated form of sudden death, is a right ventricular disease.[3,12,15]

The action potential of M cells prolongs disproportionately relative to the action potential of other ventricular myocardial cells in response to a slowing of rate and/or in response to action potential duration (APD)-prolonging agents. The ionic basis for these features of the M cell may include the presence of a smaller slowly activating delayed rectifier current (I_{Ks}), a larger late sodium current (late I_{Na}), and a larger Na–Ca exchange current ($I_{Na–Ca}$). Larger I_{ks} in M cells isolated from the right versus left ventricles also have been described. In different species, transmural and apico-basal differences in the density of I_{Kr} channels also have been described, together with differences in Ca^{2+} channel properties between epicardial and

endocardial ventricular cells, with larger I_{ca} in endocardial than in epicardial myocytes.[3,15]

Electrophysiologically, M cells appear to be a hybrid between Purkinje and ventricular cells. Differently from epicardium and endocardium, but like Purkinje fibers, M cells show a prominent APD prolongation and develop early after depolarizations in response to I_{Kr} blockers, whereas delayed after depolarizations in response to agents that produce calcium overload in the cardiac cell. Unlike Purkinje fibers, and similar to endocardium and epicardium, M cells display an APD prolongation in response to I_{Ks} blockers. Purkinje and M cells also respond differently to α-adrenergic agonists. α1-adrenoceptor stimulation produces APD prolongation in Purkinje fibers, but abbreviation in M cells, and little or no change in endocardium and epicardium. Also, disparities in regional distribution and density of M cells within the ventricular wall have been described, with variations among different species.[3,15]

Correlation between AP Phases and QT Interval Components

The morphologic electrocardiographic characteristics of the normal ventricular repolarization; that is, the QT interval on the surface ECG (isoelectric J point and ST segment, smooth and progressive elevated T wave) results from the complex summation of different APDs between different transmural layers in different cardiac region.

J point and isoelectric ST segment
The J point is a theoretic point that in normal conditions should lie on the isoelectric line, because by definition at that J point there is no transmural gradient, as the depolarization is completed and repolarization has not started yet. During phases 1 and 2 of the cardiac action potential, the absence of difference of electrical gradient between endocardial and epicardial layers explains the isoelectrical J point and ST segment. During phase 3, the different AP durations (APD) within the ventricular wall with temporal heterogeneity among different cardiac regions explains the deviation from the isoelectric line and the subsequent onset of the T wave (see **Fig. 2**).

T wave
The genesis of the T wave is still incompletely understood. The normal upright T-wave configuration (concordant with the QRS complex) is explained by assuming that the repolarization wavefront travels in a direction opposite to depolarization. Transmural and apico-basal heterogeneity of the final phases of the AP within ventricular myocardium are thought to be

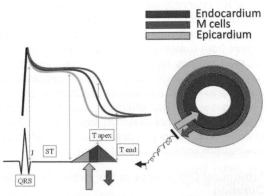

Fig. 2. Voltage gradients on either side of the midmyocardial (M) region and the inscription of the T wave.

responsible for inscription of the T wave. During phase 3, epicardial and endocardial layers have different APDs, because the epicardial repolarization occurs earlier than endocardial, generating a "transmural gradient" and a transmural current directed from the epicardium to the endocardium.

An exploring electrode on the body surface will then register a negative wavefront (ie, the repolarization wavefront) moving away from the epicardium to the endocardium, generating a positive T wave on the surface ECG.[1,2] The recording of monophasic action potentials (MAP) at multiple endocardial and epicardial sites in normal hearts have confirmed the presence of a *transmural gradient of repolarization*, with earlier repolarization occurring at the epicardium.[14] MAP recordings confirmed the presence of *inter-regional gradients*, with longer MAPs at septal and diaphragmatic sites, and shorter MAPs at anteroapical and posterolateral sites.[3]

Under normal conditions, the epicardial is the earliest to repolarize and the M cell action potential is often the last. Full repolarization of the epicardial action potential is coincident with the peak of the T wave and repolarization of the M cells coincides with the end of the T wave. Thus, the APD of the M cells usually determines the QT interval duration. The interval between the peak and end of the T wave (Tpeak − Tend) has been suggested to provide an index of the transmural dispersion of ventricular repolarization (TDR), which may be an index of proarrhythmic risk.[3,15]

U wave and QTU complex

The precise mechanisms of normal and abnormal U waves are still unknown. A distinction should be made between normal isolated U waves and abnormal QTU complexes. Originally, U wave were attributed to longer repolarization of the Purkinje network or to late depolarization of certain myocardium regions. More recent studies suggested that even normal U waves may be related to the activity of the M cells present in ventricular midmyocardium.[3,15]

The definition of abnormal U waves is the most controversial. It is possible that abnormal U waves are rather abnormal T waves fusing with U waves. Camel hump or notched T waves, with late components interrupting the descending T-wave limb often defined as QTU complexes, can be seen during several conditions of congenital or acquired prolonged repolarization. M cells have been identified as responsible for the prolongation of QT interval with abnormal T-U wave configuration on surface ECG (see **Fig. 2**). M cells have greater APD prolongation than epicardial or endocardial in response to slowing of heart rate and to agents

and conditions likely to prolong APD, and are known to play a significant role in the genesis of cardiac arrhythmias associated with afterdepolarization and triggered activity. During normal conditions, M cells are closely coupled electrically to adjacent cell layers and may not be manifest in the ECG. However, during conditions that produce electrical uncoupling from adjacent cell layers, the M cells may have profound effects on the morphology of repolarization, producing QTU complexes with bizarre configuration and prolonged duration as well as apparent prominent U waves.[3,15] The occurrence of prominent QTU complexes, with distinct gene-specific morphologic patterns of abnormal repolarization, have been described in congenital LQTS, and have been associated with increased risk of malignant arrhythmias.[9,16,17]

DYNAMICS OF VENTRICULAR REPOLARIZATION

The ventricular repolarization is a dynamic phenomenon, which is continuously modified by several physiologic modulators, including heart rate levels and autonomic nervous system activities, circadian variation, and age and gender effects.

Rate Dependence of Ventricular Repolarization

The heart rate level is the main modulator of the ventricular repolarization duration. The rate dependence of QT interval, generally defined as QT dynamicity or QT-RR relation, reflects the APD dependence on cycle length, a fundamental property of cardiac muscle. Like APD, also QT interval duration decreases at shorter cycle lengths, and prolongs at longer cycle lengths, mainly because at increasing heart rates different outward K^+ ionic currents are activated. During the phase 3 of action potential, outward delayed rectifying currents based on voltage-dependent mechanisms are activated. Within I_k currents, several components can be distinguished, based on their property to be activated in function of the heart rate levels: an ultrarapid component (I_{kur}), a rapid component (I_{kr}), and a slow component (I_{ks}). These distinctions are relevant, as at normal heart rates the rapid components (I_{kur} and I_{kr}) are prevalent, whereas at faster heart rates slow components (I_{ks}) are progressively more active, favoring an increased shortening of APD as the cycle length shortens.[5]

The QT dynamicity is modified by a variety of normal modulators, including autonomic nervous system activities, circadian variation, age and gender effects, and by several disease conditions, and it has been linked to individual-specific susceptibility to arrhythmias.[3,7,17]

The QT-RR relation is best described by an exponential relation, even if in the normal heart rate range is approximately linear. A flat QT-RR relation indicates lesser adaptation of QT interval at cycle length changes, with reduced QT shortening at shorter cycle lengths, whereas a steep QT-RR relation indicates an excessive QT prolongation at longer cycle lengths (**Fig. 3**).

The QT-RR relation can be studied by several methods, both in short-term or long-term conditions. In short-term conditions, the QT-RR relation is analyzed by modifying the cycle length by exercise, or by pacing, or by the administration of specific drugs or provocative tests such as tilt test or Valsalva test.[18–21]

On long-term conditions, the QT-RR relation is essentially analyzed during 24-hour Holter monitoring, using the spontaneous circadian variation of heart rates. The modulating effects of autonomic nervous system of QT interval can then be studied during long-term Holter monitoring, analyzing separately diurnal and nocturnal times at stable heart rates.[18]

Effect of the Autonomic Nervous Activity on QT Dynamicity

The autonomic nervous system plays a complex role in regulating the electrophysiological properties of ventricular repolarization. Vagal (or cholinergic) stimulation prolongs ventricular refractoriness, whereas sympathetic stimulation shortens refractoriness. When a vagal stimulation is performed in conditions of increased sympathetic tone, a greater prolongation of refractoriness results than with vagal stimulation alone. Changes in ventricular refractoriness can be mirrored by changes in QT interval duration of surface ECG. Parasympathetic blockade by atropine alone or in combination with propranolol shortens the QT interval, whereas propranolol alone has little effect on QT interval.

The autonomic nervous system strongly affects the rate dependence of the QT interval. The sympatho-vagal influences on the QT-RR relation can be studied by stress test or atrial pacing

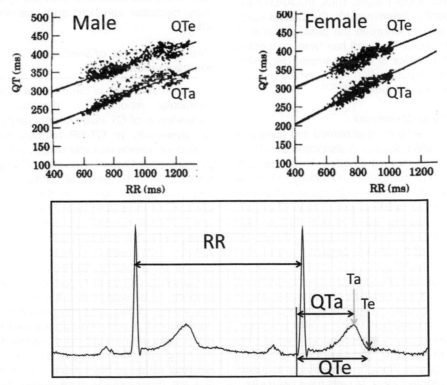

Fig. 3. QT/RR relationship in 24-hour Holter recording in healthy men and women. Each dot represents the value of QT apex (QTa) and QT end (QTe) measured for each 30-second template plotted against the corresponding RR interval. The program computed automatically both linear regressions (QTe/RR and QTa/RR) for the entire 24 hours and provided their slope, intercepts, and correlation coefficient, and mean and SD values for QTa, QTe, and RR. Note that the woman (*left*) has steeper slopes than the man (*right*), indicating that the QT interval further prolongs at longer cycle lengths.

associated to administration of specific cholinergic or sympathomimetic drugs. The slope of QT-RR relation is generally steeper during exercise stress test than during atrial pacing, suggesting that QT interval shortening at fast heart rate is increased by sympathetic stimulation. Sympathetic blockade by propranolol shows a biphasic effect on the QT-RR relation during exercise, prolonging the QT interval at long cycle lengths, and shortening the QT interval at shorter cycle lengths. In contrast, after autonomic blockade (propranolol plus atropine) the QT-RR slope is lower than in basal conditions.[18,21]

The Hysteresis Effect on QT-RR Relation

The rate adaptation of QT interval is not instantaneous, but there is a delay before a new steady state is reached. When the heart rate changes rapidly (eg, during cardiac pacing, emotional stress, abrupt initiation, or cessation of exercise), the QT interval will take longer to adapt to the new rate level.[21,22] Hysteresis is a phenomenon in which the value of a physical property (ie, the QT interval) lags behind changes in the property that affects it (the RR interval). In relation to the QT interval, the observation of "hysteresis" has been thought to represent a "memory effect" in the QT interval duration, such that the QT interval duration is affected by the direction of heart rate change (**Fig. 4**).

The mechanism of QT-RR hysteresis is not completely understood. The phenomenon is attributed to a lag in QT interval adaptation to the changes in RR interval when decreasing (exercise) versus increasing (recovery). The "hysteresis effect" in the QT-RR relationship is characterized by longer QT intervals at a given RR interval while

heart rates are increasing (RR intervals decreasing), as during exercise, and shorter QT intervals at the same RR interval when heart rates are decreasing (RR intervals increasing) during recovery. Specific alterations in autonomic tone may contribute to the hysteresis effect during exercise and recovery.[21,22]

The speed of adaptation of QT interval to a new heart rate level shows individual variations. Some individuals may have greater transient increase of QT interval during sudden heart rate changes, thus they may be particularly susceptible to arrhythmias associated with prolonged QT interval. QT-RR hysteresis may be greater in healthy subjects than in populations in which reduced parasympathetic tone has been reported, such as coronary artery disease and diabetes mellitus.[21,22]

The hysteresis phenomenon also may be at the base of the so-called "electric memory" of ventricular repolarization. Rapid ventricular pacing or an alteration of ventricular activation sequence (as in Wolff-Parkinson-White syndrome or in beats following a postextrasystolic pause) produces persistent changes in heterogeneity of repolarization and a prolongation of the QT interval (see **Fig. 4**). Ventricular electrical remodeling may be responsible for "T-wave memory," which is observed commonly in patients after periods of altered activation sequence (eg, chronic pacing). These changes have been associated with alterations of potassium currents, specifically I_{to}, implying that electrical remodeling is heterogeneously expressed in the different cell types across the transmural wall. Remodeling of gap junctions may play a prominent role in action potential changes during remodeling. Electrical remodeling of the heart takes place in response to both functional (altered electrical activation) and structural (including heart failure and myocardial infarction) stressors. These electrophysiological changes produce an unstable substrate that is prone to malignant ventricular arrhythmias. Several methods have been proposed to evaluate the instability of ventricular repolarization in clinical condition, and among them the most established are "microvolt T-wave alternans" (**Fig. 5**) and "QT Variability Index" (QTVI).

Circadian Variation of Ventricular Repolarization

Circadian changes in ventricular repolarization dynamicity have been consistently reported.[18,23,24] QT interval duration increases during sleep, independently of heart rate levels, suggesting that in physiologic conditions parasympathetic activity (or withdrawal of sympathetic activity) prolongs

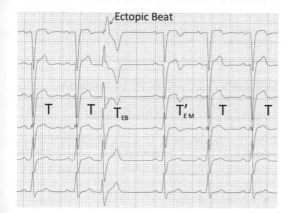

Fig. 4. QT-RR hysteresis phenomenon. The T wave of the postectopic beat shows the electric memory with a T′$_{EM}$ morphology similar to T$_{EB}$; see text for further explanation.

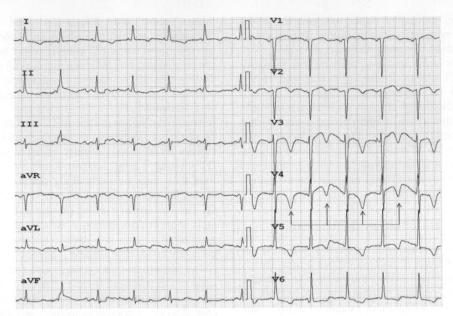

Fig. 5. ST-T wave alternans (*arrows*).

ventricular repolarization and QT interval duration. The slope QT-RR relation is also flatter during sleep, suggesting that increased parasympathetic activity (or withdrawal of sympathetic activity) reduces the rate dependency of QT interval.[18,21,25]

Preliminary data suggest that patients with coronary artery disease, when compared with healthy subjects, may show lack of circadian modulation of QT dynamicity. Also, several drugs or genetic cardiac ion channel abnormalities may modify the circadian pattern of QT dynamicity. The evaluation of the circadian modulation of QT dynamicity may have great clinical relevance, as abnormal circadian patterns of prolonged QT interval may be associated with an increased incidence of malignant arrhythmias and sudden death.[18]

Age and Gender Effect on QT Interval Duration and QT Dynamicity

Surface ECG indices of myocardial repolarization demonstrate a complex interaction between age and gender. It has long been recognized that QT interval at comparable heart rates or after correction for different heart rates (corrected QT, or QTc) is of longer duration in women compared with men (see **Fig. 3**), whereas neonates and older children do not exhibit such gender differences in the corrected QT interval.[26] Extensive ECG data indicate that the gender-related divergence in QTc interval after childhood actually reflects shortening of QTc interval in men during adolescence rather than QTc prolongation in women.[27,28] Also rate dependence of QT interval has been shown

to be gender specific, as the QT-RR relation is steeper in women than in men, due to longer QT at longer cycle lengths in women than in men.[24]

The mechanisms responsible for age-sex differences in QTc duration are still unknown. Sex hormones may contribute to QT interval shortening in men or to lack of shortening in women. Androgens may blunt QT interval prolongation to exogenous agents like quinidine. In contrast, estrogens may modify the expression of ion channels, and specifically potassium currents, at least in rat uterus, whereas estradiol may have an acute dose-dependent blocking effect on I_{ks}.[28,29] These findings may explain why women are more susceptible to the development of torsade de pointes in various settings of QT prolongation.[6,7] It remains unclear whether such relative gender differences in adults reflect an intrinsically greater tendency in women to develop torsade de pointes or whether men have some protective factor.

MORPHOLOGIC ASPECTS OF NORMAL VENTRICULAR REPOLARIZATION ON SURFACE ELECTROCARDIOGRAM

The QT interval, from Q wave onset to T wave offset, represents the time taken for ventricular depolarization and repolarization, whereas the repolarization spans between the J point to the end of the T wave (**Fig. 6**).

J Point and Early Repolarization

The J point is defined as the junction of the QRS offset with the beginning of ST segment, and it

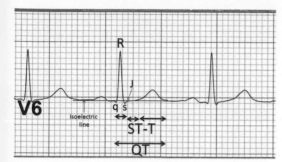

Fig. 6. Normal ventricular repolarization on surface ECG: morphologic aspects.

normally lies on the isoelectric line. The J point elevation, or early repolarization (ER) pattern, initially described as elevation of the ST segment of ≥1 lead on the 12-lead ECG, has long been considered a benign phenomenon. ER is more frequent in black individuals, men, younger individuals (age <40 years), and athletes.[29] Several studies have demonstrated associations between ER and cardiac and arrhythmic mortality.[11,14,30,31]

Several heterogeneous definitions of ER, including J point elevation and QRS complex notching or slurring, with or without concomitant ST-segment elevation have been used. The recent scientific statement from the American Heart Association attempted a standardization, proposing the definition of ER as an umbrella term including any of the following (**Fig. 7**):

- ST-segment elevation in absence of chest pain
- Terminal QRS slurring
- Terminal QRS notching[30]

Abnormal ER patterns include the Brugada patterns, a complex of ST-segment abnormalities, including downward coved and saddleback ST-segment elevations. Such patterns were defined in the BrS consensus statement and are located in precordial leads V1 through V3[12,14] (**Fig. 8**).

Another abnormal ER pattern is the Epsilon wave **Fig. 9**, a low-frequency terminal QRS deflection present in the anteroseptal precordial leads in patients with arrhythmogenic right ventricular cardiomyopathy. Its morphology can be variable but often is a broad, low-amplitude terminal QRS notch.[30]

ST Segment

The *ST segment* starts at the J point and ends at the beginning of the T wave and has a duration of 80 to 120 ms (see **Fig. 6**). The ST segment is normally on the isoelectric line, but deflections from the isoelectric line (both elevation and depression) can be present in 1 or more leads even in healthy subjects. The most important

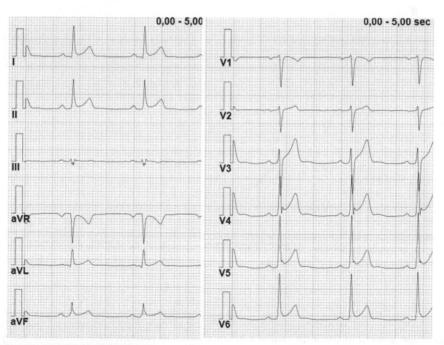

Fig. 7. Benign early repolarization pattern.

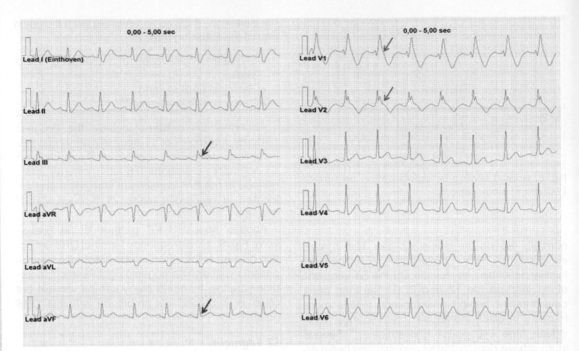

Fig. 8. J syndrome. Abnormal ER patterns include both the Brugada patter in V_1 and V_2 and malignant ER in inferior leads. The red arrows are pointing to the abnormal ER pattern with elevated J waves (more evident in V1-V2 and inferior leads, *blue arrows*).

cause of ST segment abnormality (either elevation or depression) is myocardial ischemia or infarction, but several other acquired and congenital conditions, including cardiac and noncardiac diseases and drugs may affect the ST configuration (**Box 1**).

ST elevation may have either concave, convex, or obliquely straight morphology. The most common normal variant is the so-called "benign ER pattern" characterized by mild ST elevation with tall T waves mainly in the precordial leads, more frequent in young, healthy male patients (see

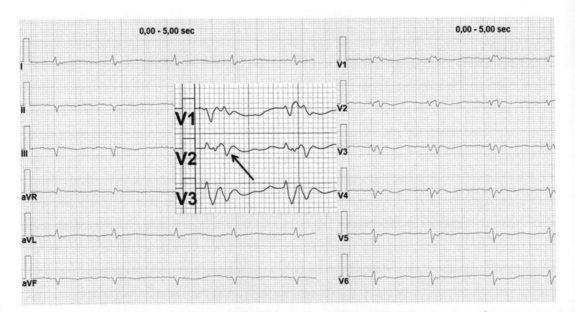

Fig. 9. Epsilon wave (*arrow*): arrhythmogenic right ventricular cardiomyopathy/dysplasia. Low-frequency terminal QRS deflection present in the anteroseptal precordial leads in patients with ventricular tachycardias (see Fig. 21 in Roberto De Ponti and colleagues' article, "General Approach to a Wide QRS Complex," in this issue.)

Box 1
Causes of ST segment abnormalities

Causes of ST Segment Elevation

- Acute myocardial infarction (ST-elevation myocardial infarction [STEMI])
- Coronary vasospasm (Printzmetal angina)
- Pericarditis
- Benign early repolarization
- Left bundle branch block
- Left ventricular hypertrophy
- Ventricular aneurysm
- Brugada syndrome
- Ventricular paced rhythm
- Raised intracranial pressure
- Pulmonary embolism and acute cor pulmonale
- Acute aortic dissection (causing inferior STEMI due to right coronary artery dissection)
- Hyperkalemia
- Sodium channel blocking drugs (secondary to QRS widening)
- J waves (hypothermia, hypercalcemia)
- Post electrical cardioversion
- Others: cardiac tumor, myocarditis, pancreas or gallbladder disease

Causes of ST Depression

- Myocardial ischemia/non-STEMI
- Reciprocal change in STEMI
- Posterior myocardial infarction
- Digoxin effect
- Hypokalemia
- Supraventricular tachycardia
- Right bundle branch block
- Right ventricular hypertrophy
- Left bundle branch block
- Left ventricular hypertrophy
- Ventricular paced rhythm

Fig. 7). The ST changes are probably linked to vagal hyperactivity, and they may be more prominent at slower heart rates and disappear in the presence of tachycardia.

T Wave

The T wave is the deflection following each QRS complex, and generally has a smooth and rounded profile, progressively rising from the ST segment, with the ascending slope generally less steep than the corresponding descending slope (see **Fig. 6**). In healthy adults, in limb leads, the T-wave axis is generally concordant with the QRs axis, as it is generally positive in leads 1 and 2 (and aVL), whereas it can be either positive or negative in lead 3 and aVF, and generally negative in aVR (particularly in women), with an amplitude less than 0.5 mV (<5 mm). In precordial leads, the T wave is generally positive (upright) in all precordial leads except V1 (particularly in women), with an amplitude less than 1.5 mV (<15 mm). A positive tall T wave in V1 (with discordant QRS complex) is almost invariably pathologic.

Normal variants of the T wave morphology are inverted T waves or bifid in the right precordial leads (V1-V3) in children, representing the dominance of right ventricular forces, often associated with bifid T-wave morphology (**Fig. 10**). Occasionally T-wave inversions in the right precordial leads may persist into adulthood and are most commonly seen in young women.[1,2]

U Wave and QTU Complex

Normal U waves are low-amplitude positive waves less than 1.5 mm tall (<0.15 mV) and 160 to 200 ms duration, that are present in many normal hearts. Normal U waves are best seen in leads V2 or V3, which are closer to the ventricular mass, then small amplitude signals may be best seen in those leads. Prominent U waves are common in bradycardia and in hypertensive patients, where they may be a normal response. Normal U-wave amplitude is generally less than 25% the T-wave amplitude, and larger U waves are generally abnormal. Criteria for abnormal U wave or QTU complex include an amplitude ≥5 mm or a U wave that is as tall or taller as the T wave that immediately precedes it. The peak of the U wave must be separated by the T-wave peak by at least 150 ms, otherwise the second wave must be interpreted as a second component of a bifid T wave or TU complex, and the measurement of the QT interval must include this late component of the T wave[3,15] (**Fig. 11**).

MEASUREMENT OF QT INTERVAL ON SURFACE-RESTING ELECTROCARDIOGRAM

Even if the simple measurement of QT interval from standard ECG tracings has the potential to identify patients at risk of ventricular tachyarrhythmias and sudden death, the QT measurement is often neglected in clinical practice.

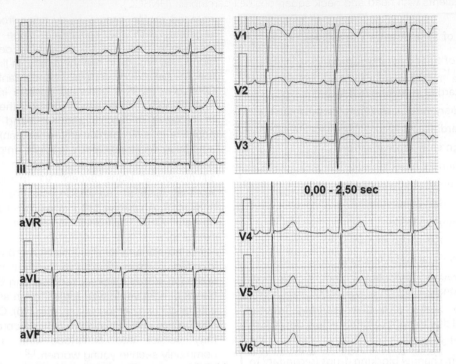

Fig. 10. Bifid T wave in V1–V3: healthy 8-year-old child.

The main problems limiting the routine measurement of QT interval are as follows:

1. The absence of univocal criteria for the determination of T-wave offset, especially when there is a partial superimposition of T and U waves
2. The absence of general consensus on the best formula for adjusting QT interval by heart rate
3. The insufficient diffusion of appropriate age-related and gender-related normal values for corrected QT intervals
4. The still prevalent use of ECG analysis made on paper printouts, which does not allow precise and fast automatic analysis, and limits the creation of a large digital database for easy serial comparison among consecutive tracings

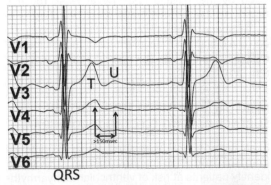

Fig. 11. Normal U wave and QTU complex (see text for details).

The QT interval duration can be derived either from the *standard 12-lead ECG tracing*, or from *continuous ECG monitoring* obtained at rest or during special procedures (such as exercise stress test or cardiac pacing), or from *long-term Holter monitoring*. The QT interval duration can be obtained either by *manual* (visual) or by *automatic* (computerized) method.

Methods to Calculate QT Duration from Standard Resting Electrocardiogram

The standard 12-lead ECG tracing at 25 mm/s paper speed at 10 mm/mV amplitude is generally adequate for accurate measurement of QT interval duration. Faster paper speed (50 mm/s) does not provide significant advantages, because it makes it more difficult to define the morphology of repolarization waveforms, especially low-amplitude waves, such as U waves.

Conventionally, the QT interval is measured in lead II. When the QT interval cannot be measured in lead II, the best alternative leads are aVR, aVF, V5, V6, and V4, in that sequence. It differs maximally from that in leads II and aVL.[32–36]

The vast majority of QT analysis is still performed on paper printouts, either directly on paper copies or with the support of on-screen caliper methods applied to the scanned tracing. The QT interval can be obtained by *visual determination on paper tracings*, by the aid of a caliper, with an accuracy level of 20 to 40 ms (resolution corresponding to 1 small box, equivalent to 40 ms at 25 mm/s paper speed). More accurate and reproducible measurements can be achieved by using a *digitizing pad* with an accuracy level of 5 ms.

More recently, the QT measurements are obtained by new methods of *digital conversion of paper ECGs into waveforms*, which allows the conversion of an image of paper ECG, obtained by scanning the paper ECG into a digital format. By this software, paper ECGs are converted into true digital ECGs and it will then be possible to process these ECGs as if they were originally acquired in digital format. This *combined manual and computer approach* provides high-quality ECG data, and it is highly recommended at core laboratories performing centralized analyses of large ECG database (eg, clinical trials or studies to evaluate the effect of certain drugs on different ECG parameters).[37]

Several current 12-lead digital ECG recorders now include *computer algorithms for automatic measurement* of several ECG parameters. Automatic measurements of RR and QRS intervals are generally accurate, as the R spikes are high-frequency waveforms, whereas automatic measurements of QT interval, including low-frequency T and U waveforms, are often less reliable, particularly in abnormal tracings with complex T and U wave morphology.[38]

Criteria to Define the T Wave End

The principal difficulty when measuring QT interval is the definition of T wave end, particularly when there is partial superimposition of T and U waves. Different methods can lead to quite different results, above all in presence of abnormal T-wave configuration. The oldest and more widely used method, proposed by Lepeshkin and Surawicz,[33] is to draw a *tangent to the steepest point of the downslope of the T wave*, and to consider as T-wave offset the crossing of the tangent with the isoelectric line (**Fig. 12**). This method can

adequately measure QT interval duration both on standard 12-lead ECG tracing, and on ECG recording taken during exercise stress test or pacing, or during long-term Holter monitoring, and can be applied both by visual and automatic determination, provided that a stable isoelectric line can be determined. However, this method may *underestimate the real duration of ventricular repolarization*, because it ignores the late components in abnormal T-wave configuration (diphasic or "camel" T wave or prominent U wave inscribed in the T wave).

To overcome the limitations of the tangent method, Campbell and colleagues[34] proposed to define the *T wave end as the return to the TP baseline*. When a U wave interrupted the T wave before the return to baseline, the QT interval was measured to the *nadir* of the curve between T and U waves. Biphasic T waves were measured to the time of final return to baseline. This method probably reflects more accurately the real duration of the ventricular repolarization in the entire myocardium, but it introduces a *large degree of subjectivity*, particularly when diphasic T waves are present or when large U waves interrupt the return of the T wave to the baseline. This method can be effectively applied to visual measurements (after an adequate training of the operator to assure consistency of the results), but it is less suitable to be implemented in computer algorithms for automatic measurements, as it requires the definition of a given threshold for the amplitude below which T-wave or U-wave potentials return to baseline. Another method proposed by Laguna and colleagues,[39] mainly for computerized measurements applied to Holter monitoring, automatically defines the T wave end on a beat-to-beat basis, by calculating the first derivative of the ECG signal and comparing it with a threshold value.

Additional Parameters of Ventricular Repolarization

Beside total QT interval duration from Q wave offset to T wave end (QTend or QTe), several parameters have been proposed to characterize different aspects of ventricular repolarization. Some measures are already used in clinical routine, whereas others are still investigational.

T wave peak
Because the T wave peak (Tp, or T wave apex, Ta) can be more accurately identified than T wave end, both by manual and by automatic measurements, it has been proposed to measure the interval from Q wave onset to T wave peak (QTp) as an alternative to the total QT interval duration to the T wave

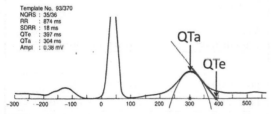

Template No. 93/370
NQRS : 35/36
RR : 874 ms
SDRR : 18 ms
QTe : 397 ms
QTa : 304 ms
Ampl : 0.38 mV

QTa

QTe

-300 -200 -100 0 100 200 300 400 500

Fig. 12. Criteria to define the T wave end and apex tangent to the steepest point of the downslope of the T wave, and to consider as T wave offset the crossing of the tangent with the isoelectric line.

end (QTe) (see **Figs. 2** and **3**). The T wave peak is the point of maximal T-wave amplitude, and it can be determined automatically by fitting a parabola through the samples of a windows following the QRS complex.[19,38] However, QTp should not be considered equivalent to the total QT duration (QTe), particularly in prolonged QT syndromes, where the QT prolongation may affect specifically the terminal components of the T wave.[3,12]

Terminal late repolarization

The duration of the terminal components of the T wave can be measured from the T wave peak to the T wave end (*TpTe*).[3,12] An increased duration of the terminal portion of the T wave may reflect an *increased TDR*, defined as the difference in APD between different myocardial layers (endocardial, midmyocardial or M cells, and epicardial cells), which might be associated with increased propensity to reentrant arrhythmias. Few clinical studies have so far used this parameter. Although QTp interval is strongly dependent on heart rate, TpTe interval is less rate-dependent, suggesting that autonomic modulation mainly affects the early phase of ventricular repolarization, whereas the terminal phase is mainly determined by the intrinsic properties of cardiac myocites.[3,19,38]

QT dispersion

The QT interval duration varies across the different ECG leads, and it is generally longer in anterior precordial leads (V2-V3), probably reflecting temporal and spatial regional variation in the ventricular repolarization process. The difference of QT duration among the different ECG leads is defined as *QT dispersion* **Fig. 13**. Increased QT dispersion may indicate increased heterogeneity within the heart, which may favor arrhythmogenesis.[40,41]

There is little or no sex difference in QT dispersion, and age-related differences, if present, appear to be small (<10 ms). The need for a heart rate–corrected QT (QTc) dispersion has not been conclusively established. Reported values of QT dispersion vary widely, ranging from 10 to 71 ms in healthy subjects (mean 33 ms; median 37 ms).[41] Large studies and literature reviews suggested that the upper normal limit of QT dispersion in healthy subjects is 65 ms, whereas other reports claim that QT dispersion greater than 40 ms was the best cutoff for predicting the inducibility of sustained ventricular tachycardia during an electrophysiology study.[40,41]

Formula to Evaluate the Rate Dependence of QT Interval

To ascertain that changes in QT interval actually represent changes in ventricular repolarization, rather than simply changes in heart rate, the QT interval must be corrected to account for heart rate variations. Several formulas have been proposed to express the heart rate dependence of QT interval and to compare QT intervals obtained at different cycle lengths.[32,33,42] The different equations normalize the QT interval obtained at a given cycle length to the value that it would have had at a rate of 60 beats per minute (or 1000 ms RR interval). Standard rate-correction formulas apply only to the field of resting ECG, whereas during non–steady-state conditions, the use of these formulas is generally inadequate.[36,43]

Rate-correction formula

The 4 major correction formulas are illustrated in **Table 1**. The earliest and most widely used is the *Bazett square-root formula*, where rate-corrected QT interval (QTc) is calculated from the QT divided by the square root of the preceding RR (in seconds).[32] The Bazett formula has been criticized because of its inaccuracy and overcorrection at

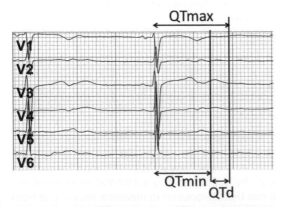

Fig. 13. QT dispersion: patient with acquired QT long syndrome.

Table 1 Correction formula for rate-adjusted QT interval	
Name of the Formula	**Correction Formula**
Bazett	$QT_c = QT/\sqrt{RR}$
Fridericia	$QT_f = QT/\sqrt[3]{RR}$
Linear	$QT_l = QT + a(1-RR)$
Exponential	$QT_e = QT - be^{-k1000} - e^{-kRR}$
Prediction	$QTp \ (ms) = 65.600/(100 + heart\ rate)$

high and low heart rates. Much less used is the *Fridericia cubit-root formula,* which has the same limitations as the Bazett formula. Among the *linear formulas,* the most popular is the Framingham Heart Study based on a population of 5018 subjects.[34] The most accepted *exponential formula* was proposed by Ashman, and later confirmed by Sarma, on the basis of several clinical and experimental studies.[42] Although exponential formulas fit many biological processes closely, in this case they give too low QT values at low heart rate.[36,43] Of note, in resting conditions *most formulas provide almost equivalent results.* Even if the rate dependence of QT interval is probably best described by an exponential relation, in the normal heart rate range, the QT-RR relation is approximately linear.[18,19,24,33]

The rate dependence of QT interval varies with sex and age. The rate-corrected QT interval duration measured at standard 12-lead ECG is similar by gender in infancy and childhood, and decreases in healthy men but not in women.[26,28,32] Although blunted, gender differences are still present in elderly subjects, in whom longer QTc values are associated with increased cardiac mortality.[27,44,45]

Nowadays the most common QT interval correction, generally utilized in clinical practice, is the Bazett's Formula.[32] Over the years, a large experience has been later accumulated, and today the upper limits for normal values by Bazett's formula are considered 440 msec for adult males and children below age 15 years, and 460 msec for adult women. These normal limits apply only to resting standard ECG, and should not be considered as normative for other applications, such as measurements of circadian QTc variability during Holter monitoring or QTc variation during exercise stress test.[36]

Predicted QT interval

An alternative approach to rate-correction formula is to calculate a predicted QT interval (QTp) as proposed by Rautaharju and colleagues.[26] This method does not use a rate-correction formula, and is particularly useful to define a limit for short QT intervals, as the Bazett formula tends to underestimate QTc at lower heart rates and overestimates QTc at higher heart rates. The QTp formula, derived from investigating the QT interval in 14,379 healthy individuals, computed the predicted QT interval as QTp (ms) = 65.600 / (100 + heart rate). In this study, the prevalence of QT interval shorter than 88% of QTp (QT/QTp <88%, equivalent to 2 SD below the mean) was 2.5%, thus a QT interval less than 88% of QTp (2 SD below mean predicted value) at a particular heart rate might be considered as the lower limit of

normal. At a heart rate of 60 beats per minute, a normal QTp would be 410 ms and 88% of QTp would be 360 ms. Thus, a QT interval (not QTc) value of ≤360 ms at heart rate of 60 beats per minute might reasonably be considered to be a shorter than normal QT interval.

MEASUREMENTS OF QT DYNAMICITY AND QT VARIABILITY

Repolarization dynamics and variability are of increasing interest as exercise-induced or Holter-derived parameters reflecting changes in myocardial vulnerability and contributing to increased risk of arrhythmic events and sudden death. *QT dynamicity* is usually defined as the phenomenon describing and quantifying QT adaptation to changing heart rate, whereas *QT variability* reflects beat-to-beat changes in repolarization duration and morphology and such changes can be quantified using several algorithms currently in various phases of development and validation.

The measurement of QT interval from ambulatory Holter monitoring requires computerized automatic procedures, with specific technical problems, due to relatively low sampling rates, shifting of the isoelectric baseline, low signal-to-noise ratio, and difficult determination of T wave end at fast heart rates. Reliable long-term automatic measurements from Holter monitoring can be obtained by *averaging procedures* that generate a low-noise ECG signal. Averaging procedures require the alignment of several consecutive beats over a given time interval with respect to the R-wave peak, generally estimated by parabolic interpolation. Averaged ECG templates are then analyzed by specific algorithms that automatically detect QRS and T-wave features. Averaging methods generally provide *robust QT interval measurements,* but they ignore the instantaneous variations in QT duration in function of cycle length changes. In contrast, *beat-to-beat analysis* can explore the *instantaneous fluctuations of QT duration* as function of cycle length changes. Long-term beat-to-beat QT analysis often requires the removal of a large proportion of nonphysiologic data due to noise. Beat-to-beat QT analyses are best applied to short-term high-quality ECG recordings obtained in controlled conditions.

Several methodological approaches have been proposed to evaluate the long-term QT dynamicity and variability during long-term Holter monitoring. Some of those methods have been implemented on different commercial Holter systems, becoming available for routine clinical use. Altered QT dynamicity and increased QT variability were observed in several conditions with increased risk of arrhythmias. However, more studies are needed to define the potential clinical usefulness for risk stratification purposes of QT dynamicity and QT variability methods, and compare these methods with exercise-induced T-wave alternans.[20,45,46]

Circadian Pattern of Rate-Corrected QT Interval

The circadian pattern of QT interval dynamicity can be evaluated from 24-hour ECG Holter recordings by automatic QT interval measures, based on averaging or beat-to-beat analysis, and the measured QT is then rate-adjusted by one of the formulas described previously, generally the Bazett. The algorithms generally provide the means and range of the QT and QTc interval and allows the identification of *peaks of prolonged QTc interval*; that is, the proportion of QTc intervals above a given threshold (eg, QTc >500 ms). Abnormal circadian patterns of prolonged QT interval may be associated with an increased incidence of malignant arrhythmias.[32] Also, several drugs or genetic cardiac ion channel abnormalities may modify the circadian pattern of QT variability.[8,32] Therefore, the possibility to identify abnormalities of the circadian QT variability by automatic noninvasive procedures has potential large applications in clinical practice.

Long-Term Evaluation of QT-RR Relation

The rate dependence of QT interval can be evaluated from ECG Holter recordings by computing the regression between QT intervals and correspondent RR intervals, both on the entire 24-hour or on preselected time periods (eg, day vs night time) (see **Fig. 3**). When considering a *linear relation*, in general, a *steep slope* of the QT-RR relation indicates a strong rate dependence of the QT interval, with further prolongation at longer cycle lengths, and adequate shortening at shorter cardiac cycles; in contrast, a *flat slope* indicates that the QT interval is less dependent from the cardiac cycle, and it fails to shorten at shorter cycles. Of note, the QTa-RR relation is generally steeper than the QTe-RR relation, suggesting that the QTa interval is more rate-dependent than QTe, suggesting that *autonomic modulation mainly affects the early phase of ventricular repolarization*.[19,24] The QT-RR relation shows typical *day-night differences*,[18] with flatter slope during night than during day-time. Also, the QT-RR relation is steeper in healthy women than in healthy men, in parallel with a longer duration of the corrected QT interval observed in women.[24] So far, normal values for rate dependence of QT interval are based on small-scale studies, and larger studies are necessary to obtain appropriate reference

values to be used for prognostic risk stratification. Based on the available data, mean QTa/RR slope is 0.20 ± 0.04 in women and 0.16 ± 0.03 in men (normal range 0.09–0.28), and mean QTe/RR slope is 0.16 ± -0.04 in women and 0.13 ± 0.03 in men (normal range 0.08–0.24).[24] The QT-RR relation can be impaired in conditions of congenital and acquired prolonged ventricular repolarization, and abnormal patterns of rate adaptation of QT interval have been observed in conditions of prolonged ventricular repolarization, including congenital LQTS and drug-induced long QT. Increased QT–R-R slopes were also observed in conditions at risk for ventricular arrhythmias, as ischemic and nonischemic cardiomyopathies.[20]

Noteworthy, the patterns of the QT-RR relation were shown to be very different among healthy individuals, and very often the QT-RR relation was best expressed by regressions different from the linear regression, such as parabolic or exponential regression. Therefore, for detailed precise studies of the QTc interval (for example, drug-induced QT interval prolongation), the individual QT-RR relation has to be taken into account.[44]

QT Variability Index

The QTVI is a noninvasive measure of repolarization lability that has been applied to a wide variety of subjects with cardiovascular disease. It is a ratio of normalized QT variability to normalized heart rate variability, including an assessment of autonomic nervous system tone. The approach assesses beat-to-beat variability in the duration of the QT and U wave in conventional surface electrocardiographic recordings, as well as determines the heart rate variability from the same recording. As opposed to T wave alternans, QTVI assesses variance in repolarization at all frequencies. Several studies have assessed the utility of QTVI in predicting VT/VF, cardiac arrest, or cardiovascular death. although the clinical utility of this index needs definitive exploration.[46,47]

Microvolt T-Wave Alternans

Microvolt-level T-wave alternans (TWA) assessed by spectral method during an exercise stress test has been widely studied for risk stratification. Several studies have documented the association of a positive TWA with total mortality and arrhythmic events. Nevertheless, the need to achieve an elevated and stabilized heart rate resulting in a considerable proportion of indeterminate test results constitutes one of the main limitations of this method. It is well recognized that arrhythmic events may be triggered not only by physical but also by mental stress and are not necessarily associated with exercise. Detection of TWA in ambulatory electrocardiogram recordings during daily activities might be a valuable option in risk stratification. The most established method is the modified moving average (MMA) technique for detection of TWA. So far, MMA-TWA has been studied in more than 5000 patients, including those evaluated during exercise as well as during daily activities with ambulatory ECG recordings. These studies indicate that increased MMA-TWA is associated with higher risk of cardiac mortality and arrhythmic events.[45,46]

CONDITIONS PROVOKING REPOLARIZATION ABNORMALITIES

Ventricular repolarization is affected by several congenital or acquired conditions, including abnormalities in ionic and hormonal levels, several cardiac and noncardiac drugs, and multiple cardiac disease, such as cardiac ischemia, cardiomyopathies, and channellopathies due to cardiac ionic gene mutations, and by many noncardiac diseases. Additional age-gender and gene-environment interactions are often required for a given factor to determine the occurrence of repolarization disturbances and arrhythmogenesis.[3,6–9,48]

Electrolyte Disturbance

Electrolyte or metabolic disturbances, including hyperkalemia and hypokalemia, hypercalcemia or hypocalcemia, and hypomagnesemia, due to renal or gastrointestinal or hormonal diseases, or to the use of diuretics, are the most common causes of perturbation of ventricular repolarization, provoking QT interval and in T wave morphology changes.

Hyperkalemia has a direct effect on some of the potassium channels by increasing their activity, provoking a faster repolarization of the cardiac action potential, with steeper phase 3, and tenting of the T waves (**Fig. 14**). In severe hyperkalemia, a very large QRS continues with a bizarre repolarization: the ST segment disappears and the QRS merges with a very short ventricular repolarization (**Fig. 15**).

Hypokalemia has almost opposite effects, as it prolonged the phase 3 of cardiac action potential, mainly by reducing I_{Kr} and I_{ks} currents. ECG

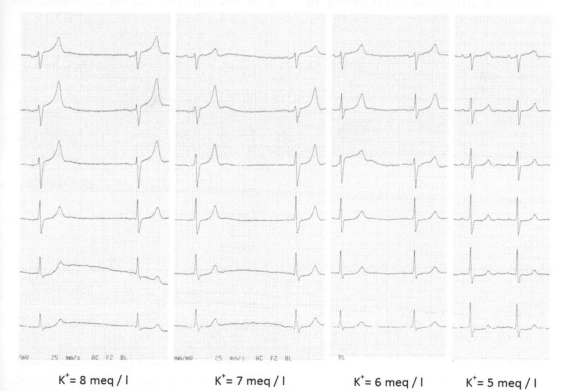

| K⁺ = 8 meq / l | K⁺ = 7 meq / l | K⁺ = 6 meq / l | K⁺ = 5 meq / l |

Fig. 14. Electrocardiographic anomalies associated with hyperkalemia: QT shortening, T-wave picking. Progressive reduction of ECG alterations during hemodialytic therapy (K + 8 ->5 mEq/L).

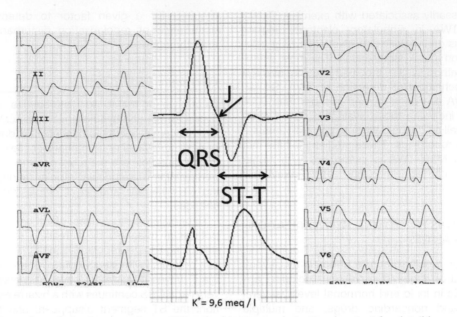

Fig. 15. Severe hyperkalemia: a very large QRS and a bizarre repolarization (see text for details).

changes associated with hypokalemia are flattened T waves, ST segment depression, and prolongation of the QT interval. U wave amplitude is slightly increased, and QTU complex may occur (**Fig. 16**).

Hypercalcemia is associated with a shortening of the ST segment, and consequently the QT interval, whereas very high Ca levels broaden the T wave and may normalize the QT interval. Vice

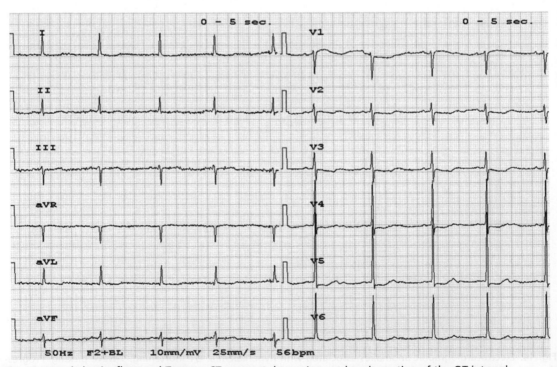

Fig. 16. Hypokalemia: flattened T waves, ST segment depression, and prolongation of the QT interval.

versa, hypocalcemia prolongs the ST segment and the QT interval and flattens the T wave.

Hypomagnesemia is often associated with other electrolyte imbalances like hypokalemia and hypocalcemia, which confound the ECG changes. In the few reported cases of isolated hypomagnesemia, global T-wave inversions and prolonged corrected QT interval were described.

Cardiac and Noncardiac Drugs

Many cardiac drugs (mainly antiarrhythmic class 1a and class 3 drugs) and noncardiac drugs (antihistamines, antipsychotics, antidepressants, neuroleptics, anesthetics, antibiotics, antimalarials, and antiprotozoal agents) have been implicated in the prolongation of the QT interval (**Fig. 17**). Virtually all QT-prolonging drugs act by blocking potassium channels, mainly the rapid component of the delayed rectifier potassium channel (I_{kr}) encoded by the human ether a go-go related gene (hERG).[6,7,48,49] Some of these drugs have shown an increased incidence of fatal polymorphic ventricular tachycardia or torsade de points (TdP). QT prolongation and proarrhythmic effects of drugs have been shown to be more frequent among women. An updated list of specific drugs

that prolong the QT interval can be found at www.qtdrugs.org (**Box 2**).

Drug-to-drug interactions have been described, as several of these drugs are metabolized by the cytochrome P450 enzymes. Gene-drug interactions may also exist at different levels: ion channel mutations may increase the risk of QT prolongation by drug use, or common genetic variants associated with longer QT interval may potentiate the QT-prolonging effect of drugs, and variation within drug metabolizing and transporting proteins that influence drug pharmacokinetics may all favor potential proarrhythmic effects of drugs.[6,7,48]

Cardiac and Noncardiac Diseases

Coronary artery disease and myocardial infarction are well known to prolong the QT interval, and the rate-adjusted QT interval (QTc) was shown to be prognostic of sudden death in patients with myocardial infarction[48,50] (**Fig. 18**). Abnormalities of ventricular repolarization have been described in patients with heart failure, hypertrophic cardiomyopathies, both primary or secondary due to arterial hypertension, and in acute (**Fig. 19**) and chronic (**Fig. 20**) acquired or idiopathic cardiomyopathies.[48]

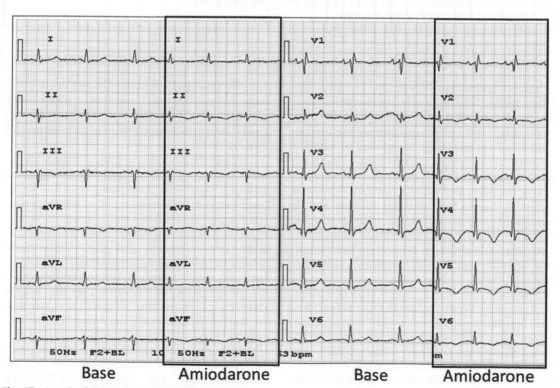

Fig. 17. Acquired QT prolongation (amiodarone).

Box 2
Cardiac and noncardiac drugs that can cause QT prolongation

Cardiac medications
- Antiarrhythmic drugs
  - Class Ia (quinidine, procainamide, disopromide)
  - Class III (dofetilide, ibutilide, sotalol, amiodarone)

Noncardiac medications
- Antihistamines (terfenadine,[a] astemizole[a])
- Antipsychotic and antidepressant agents
- Neuroleptic (haloperidol, droperidol, thioridazine, chlorpromazine)
- Atypical antipsychotics (sertindole,[a] ziprasidone, risperidone, zimeldine, citalopram)
- Antidepressants (amitriptyline, imipramine, maprotiline, doxepin, fluoxetine)
- Opiate agonists (methadone, levomethadyl)
- Anesthetic agents (sevoflurane, isoflurane)
- Antibiotics
  - Quinolone (sparfloxacin,[a] levofloxacin, moxifloxacin, grepafloxacin[a])
  - Macrolide (erythromycin, clarithromycin)
- Antimalarials (quinine, halofantrine)
- Antiprotozoal (Pentamidine)
- Antifungal (azole group)
- Antimotility agents (cisapride,[a] domperidone)
- Other (arsenic trioxide, bepridil, probucol)

Complete and updated list of drugs can be obtained from www.qtdrugs.org.
  [a] Withdrawn from market or discontinued.

Several noncardiac conditions, including diabetes mellitus, increased or lower thyroid hormone concentrations, lipid abnormalities, high body mass index, and cerebrovascular and neuromuscular diseases have been associated with abnormalities of ventricular repolarization, including prolonged QT interval.[48]

The prevalence of QT interval prolongation is higher in people with *diabetes mellitus* and its complications. Also diabetes is often associated with a spectrum of conditions, including hypertension, lipid abnormalities, autonomic neuropathy, and cardiomyopathy, all affecting ventricular repolarization.

It is well known that *thyroid hormonal disfunction* can affect ventricular conduction characteristics and duration of ventricular repolarization. Increased thyroid function is related to several factors that shorten the ventricular repolarization, such as hyperthermia, hypercalcemia, and modification of the autonomic tone. Thyroid hormones may alter conduction properties of myocardial cells by affecting the sodium pump density and enhancement of Na^+ and K^+ permeability, whereas lower levels of thyroid hormones may cause prolonged repolarization and longer QT interval.[48]

Cerebrovascular diseases and stroke are often associated with QT prolongation and T wave changes, regardless of the presence of preexisting heart disease. QT interval duration and dispersion were higher in patients with intracerebral hemorrhage as compared with infarction stroke and transient ischemic attack. The size of the lesions seems to be related to the extent of the ECG effects, as larger lesions seem to provoke larger QT prolongation and alteration of the T-wave morphology. These may be due to a higher level of catecholamines, with increased sympathetic activity.[51]

Several *neuromuscular diseases* are associated with abnormalities of ventricular repolarization and supraventricular and ventricular arrhythmias. Among them, myotonic dystrophy type 1 (DM1),

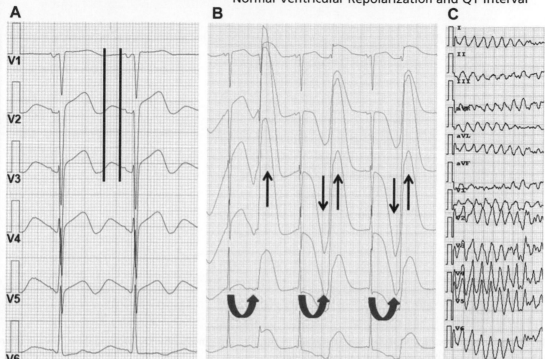

Fig. 18. Impaired ventricular repolarization (*A, B*) and ventricular fibrillation development (*C*). Impaired ventricular repolarization (*A, B*) and ventricular fibrillation (*C*) development in a patient with myocardial ischemia. Ventricular fibrillation is preceded by extreme QT prolongation and ventricular dispersion (*A*); therefore, ventricular extrasystolic bigeminism with global alternans of ventricular repolarization. The straight arrows (*B*) indicate the alternans in the T wave polarity, while the curved arrows indicate the alternans in the T wave amplitude during ventricular bigeminism.

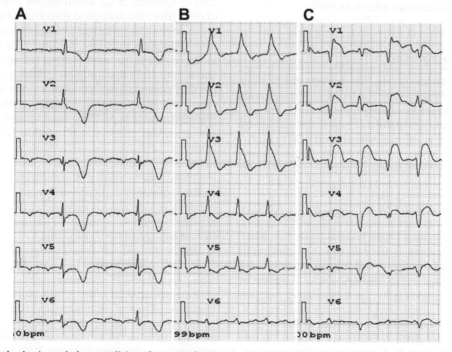

Fig. 19. Arrhythmia and abnormalities of ventricular repolarization in acute myocarditis: during the first 3 days of the disease, the patient developed atrium ventricular block with QT prolongation (*A*), then a "Brugada-like" pattern (*B*), and finally an intraventricular conduction delay with ST elevation in precordial leads (*C*).

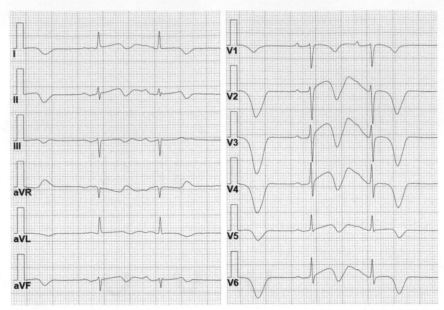

Fig. 20. Abnormalities of ventricular repolarization in chronic cardiomyopathy: QT prolongation, T-wave alternans, and deep negative T wave in the precordial leads.

an autosomal dominant neuromuscular disorder associated with various cardiac rhythm disturbances, was demonstrated to carry a missplicing of SCN5A, a gene implicated in BrS, and higher prevalence of Brugada pattern has been described in patients with DM1.[52,53]

Genetic Background

Mutations of the genes that encode the protein ionic channels (mainly I_{Kr}, I_{Ks}, I_{k1}, and I_{Na}) can result in congenital channelopathies.

More than 11 different types of congenital LQTSs have been recognized, and LQT1, LQT2, and LQT3 account for most of the cases. In general, loss-of-function of potassium conductance leads to action potential prolongation.[8–10,54]

- LQT1 is caused by mutations in the KVLQT1 (or KCNQ1) gene, encoding I_{ks}. LQT1 carriers usually have a broad T-wave base (**Fig. 21**).
- LQT2 is caused by a variety of mutations in hERG potassium channel gene (KCNH2), encoding I_{kr}. LQT2 carriers show T waves of low amplitude with high incidence of notches (**Fig. 22**).
- LQT3 is caused by mutations in the sodium channel gene (SCN5A), which alters Na+ channel (I_{Na}) inactivation, inducing prolonged cardiac action potential and increased cellular excitability. LQT3 carriers frequently

have extended ST segment with relatively narrow peaked T wave (**Fig. 23**).

The "*J-wave syndromes,*" both BrS and early repolarization syndromes (ERSs), are due to a gain-of-function of I_{to}, which results in shortening of APD. This may be due to a loss-of-function mutation in SCN5A, resulting in a I_{Na} reduction. The main difference between BrS and ERS is related to the region of the ventricle most affected: in patients with BrS, accentuated J waves and fragmented potentials are observed in the epicardial region of the right ventricular outflow tract (**Fig. 24**), whereas in ERS, accentuated J waves are observed only in the inferior wall of left ventricle.[11,12]

The SQTS is much rarer and it has been related to either hyperfunction of the delayed rectifier potassium currents or hypofunction of the calcium currents, resulting in a shortening of the repolarization period and an increase in transmural dispersion of repolarization[13] (**Fig. 25**).

Also in the general normal population, the QT interval is a quantitative trait with approximately 30% heritability.[48] Common genetic variants associated with QT interval duration have been identified. Several of these are located within genes known for LQTS (KCNQ1, KCNH2 (hERG), SCN5A, KCNE1). Five percent to 20% of patients with drug-induced TdP have mutations in genes causing LQTS. These patients have a normal to borderline QTc interval at

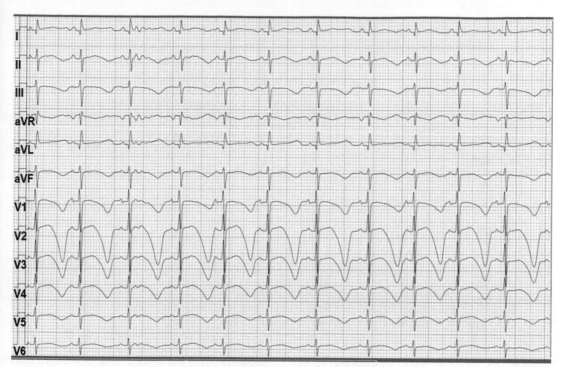

Fig. 21. LQT1 Syndrome. An 8-year-old girl with previous recurrent syncope.

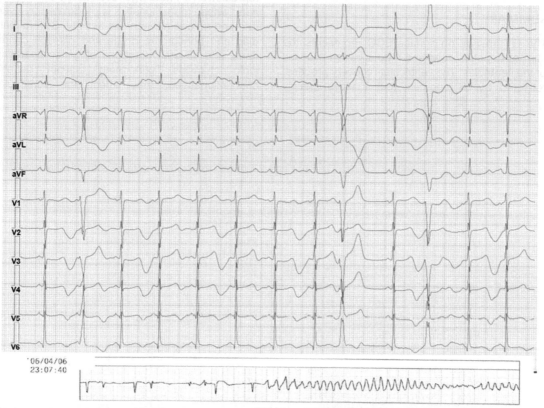

Fig. 22. LQT2 Syndrome. A 45-year-old woman who experienced recurrent syncopal episodes (TdP in the lower panel).

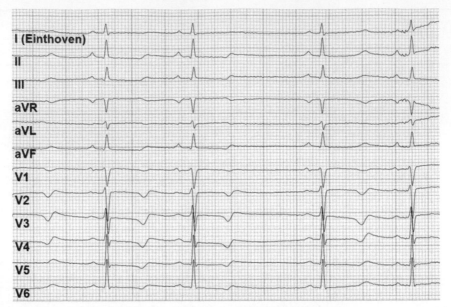

Fig. 23. LQT3 Syndrome. Typical pattern in an asymptomatic 55-year-old woman.

baseline but become more susceptible to QT prolongation and TdP when exposed to some drugs.[48]

SUMMARY

The QT interval on surface ECG represents the sum of depolarization and repolarization process of the ventricles. The ventricular recovery process, reflected by ST segment and T wave, mainly depends on the transmembrane outward transport of potassium ions to reestablish the endocellular electronegativity. Outward potassium channels represent a very heterogeneous family of ionic carriers, whose global kinetics is modulated by heart rate and autonomic nervous activity. Several cardiac and noncardiac drugs and disease conditions, and several mutations of genes encoding ionic channels, generating distinct genetic channellopathies, may affect the ventricular

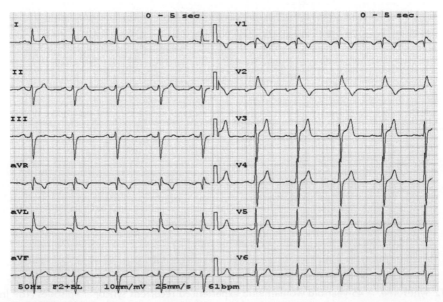

Fig. 24. Typical pattern of BrS.

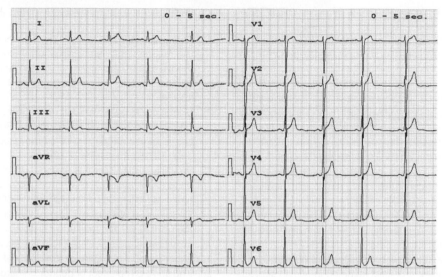

Fig. 25. SQTS.

repolarization and increase the susceptibility to ventricular arrhythmias.

The simple measurement of QT interval from surface ECG can provide a valuable marker for the identification of patients at risk of ventricular arrhythmias. However, the routine measurement of QT interval requires the use of precise and univocal criteria for the determination of T-wave offset, especially when there is a partial superimposition of T and U waves. Automatic QT interval measurements should always be taken with great care, particularly in cases of abnormal T-wave configuration. Also, QT interval must be adjusted for heart rate level, and different normal values for age and gender must be considered for diagnostic purposes.

Prolonged ventricular repolarization, with abnormal configuration and increased dispersion of QT interval duration, has been associated with an increased risk of malignant arrhythmias in congenital and acquired conditions. The Q-T interval is modulated by multiple factors, such as heart rate level, circadian rhythm, and autonomic nervous system activity, which cannot be fully evaluated by brief ECG baseline tracings. Several cardiac and noncardiac drugs and disease conditions, including cardiac gene mutation, interplay with normal modulators favoring QT prolongation and arrhythmogenesis.

The automatic computerized analysis of the long-term QT interval dynamicity and variability, particularly by Holter techniques, may provide a sort of "noninvasive electrophysiological test," exploring the interactions among triggers, autonomic nervous system, and myocardial substrate, and contributing to identify patients at high risk of malignant arrhythmias in congenital and acquired prolonged ventricular repolarization.

REFERENCES

1. Van Dam RT, Durrer D. The T wave and ventricular repolarization. Am J Cardiol 1964;14:294–300.
2. Noble D, Cohen I. The interpretation of the T wave of the electrocardiogram. Cardiovasc Res 1978;12:13–27.
3. Antzelevitch C. Ionic, molecular, and cellular bases of QT-interval prolongation and torsade de pointes. Europace 2007;9:4–15.
4. Kass RS. Delayed potassium channels in the heart: cellular, molecular and regulatory properties. In: Zipes DP, Jalife J, editors. Cardiac electrophysiology: from cell to bedside. 2nd edition. Philadelphia: WB Saunders Co; 1995. p. 74–82.
5. Schmitt N, Grunnet M, Olesen SP. Cardiac potassium channel subtypes: new roles in repolarization and arrhythmias. Physiol Rev 2014;94:609–53.
6. Roden D. The long QT syndrome and torsades de pointes: basic and clinical aspects. In: El-Sherif N, Samet P, editors. Cardiac pacing and electrophysiology. Philadelphia: WB Saunders; 1991. p. 265–83.
7. Jackman WM, Friday KJ, Anderson JL, et al. The long QT syndromes: a critical review, new clinical observations and a unifying hypothesis. Prog Cardiovasc Dis 1988;31:115–72.
8. Priori SG, Barhanin J, Hauer RNW, et al. Genetic and molecular basis of cardiac arrhythmias. Eur Heart J 1999;20:174–95.
9. Schwartz PJ, Crotti L, Insolia R. Long QT syndrome: from genetics to management. Circ Arrhythm Electrophysiol 2012;5:868–77.

10. Priori SG, Wilde AA, Horie M, et al. HRS/EHRA/ APHRS expert consensus statement on the diagnosis and management of patients with inherited primary arrhythmia syndrome. Heart Rhythm 2013;10: 287–94.

11. Brugada P, Brugada J. Right bundle branch block, persistent ST segment elevation and sudden cardiac death: a distinct clinical entity and electrocardiographic syndrome. A multicentric report. J Am Coll Cardiol 1992;20:1391–6.

12. Antzelevitch C, Yan GX, Ackerman M, et al. J-Wave syndromes expert consensus conference report: emerging concepts and gaps in knowledge. J Arrhythm 2016;32:315–39.

13. Patel C, Yan GX, Antzelevitch C. Short QT syndrome: from bench to bedside. Circ Arrhythm Electrophysiol 2010;3:401–8.

14. Franz MR, Bargheer K, Rafflenbeul W, et al. Monophasic action potential mapping in human subjects with normal electrocardiogram: direct evidence for the genesis of the T wave. Circulation 1987;75: 379–86.

15. Antzelewitch C, Sicouri S. Clinical relevance of cardiac arrhythmias generated by afterdepolarization: role of M cells in the generation of U waves, triggered activity and torsade de pointes. J Am Coll Cardiol 1994;23:259–77.

16. Moss AJ, Zareba W, Benhorin J, et al. T wave patterns in genetically distinct forms of the hereditary long QT syndrome. Circulation 1995;92:2929–34.

17. Locati ET. QT interval duration remains a major risk factor in long QT syndrome patients. J Am Coll Cardiol 2006;48:1053–5.

18. Maison-Blanche P, Catuli D, Fayn J, et al. QT interval, heart rate and ventricular arrhythmias. In: Moss AJ, Stern S, editors. Noninvasive electrocardiology: clinical aspects of Holter monitoring. London: WB Saunders Co Ltd; 1996. p. 383–404.

19. Merri M, Moss AJ, Benhorin J, et al. Relationship between ventricular repolarization and cardiac cycle length during 24-hour electrocardiographic (Holter) recordings: findings in normals and patients with long QT syndrome. Circulation 1992;85:1916–21.

20. Zareba W, Bayes de Luna A. QT dynamics and variability. Ann Noninvasive Electrocardiol 2005;10: 256–62.

21. Sundaram S, Carnethon M, Polito K, et al. Autonomic effects on QT-RR interval dynamics after exercise. Am J Physiol Heart Circ Physiol 2008;294:H490–7.

22. Pelchovitz DJ, Ng J, Chicos AB, et al. QT-RR hysteresis is caused by differential autonomic states during exercise and recovery. Am J Physiol Heart Circ Physiol 2012;302(12):H2567–73.

23. Homs E, Marti V, Guindo J, et al. Automatic measurement of corrected QT interval in Holter recordings: comparison of its dynamic behaviour in patients after myocardial infarction with and without

life-threatening arrhythmias. Am Heart J 1997;134: 181–7.

24. Stramba-Badiale M, Locati EH, Martinelli A, et al. Gender and the relationship between ventricular repolarization and cardiac cycle length during 24-hour Holter recordings. Eur Heart J 1997;18: 1000–6.

25. Molnar J, Zhang F, Weiss J, et al. Diurnal pattern of QTc interval: how long is prolonged? Possible relation to circadian triggers of cardiovascular events. J Am Coll Cardiol 1996;27:76–83.

26. Rautaharju PM, Zhou SH, Wong S, et al. Sex differences in the evolution of electrocardiographic QT interval with age. Can J Cardiol 1992;8:690–5.

27. Goldberg RJ, Bengston J, Chen ZY, et al. Duration of the QT interval and total and cardiovascular mortality in healthy persons (The Framingham Heart Study experience). Am J Cardiol 1991;67:55–8.

28. Kadish AH. The effect of gender on cardiac electrophysiology and arrhythmias. In: Zipes DP, Jalife J, editors. Cardiac electrophysiology: from cell to bedside. 2nd edition. Philadelphia: WB Saunders Co; 1995. p. 1268–75.

29. Lehmann MH, Timothy K, Frankovich D, et al. Age-sex influence on rate corrected QT interval and QT-heart rate relationship in families with genotypically characterized long QT syndrome. J Am Coll Cardiol 1997;29:93–9.

30. Patton KK, Ellinor PT, Ezekowitz M, et al, American Heart Association Electrocardiography and Arrhythmias Committee of the Council on Clinical Cardiology and Council on Functional Genomics and Translational Biology. Electrocardiographic early repolarization: a scientific statement from the American Heart Association. Circulation 2016;133: 1520–9.

31. Haïssaguerre M, Derval N, Sacher F, et al. Sudden cardiac arrest associated with early repolarization. N Engl J Med 2008;358:2016–23.

32. Bazett HC. An analysis of time relations of electrocardiograms. Heart 1920;7:353.

33. Lepeshkin E, Surawicz B. The measurement of QT interval from the electrocardiogram. Circulation 1952;6:378–88.

34. Campbell RW, Gardiner P, Amos PA, et al. Measurement of the QT interval. Eur Heart J 1985;6(Suppl D): 81–3.

35. Cowan JC, Yusoff K, Moore M, et al. Importance of lead selection in QT interval measurement. Am J Cardiol 1988;61:83.

36. Goldenberg J, Moss AJ, Zareba W. QT interval: how to measure it and what is "Normal". J Cardiovasc Electrophysiol 2006;17:333–6.

37. Badilini F, Erdem T, Zareba W, et al. ECGScan: a method for conversion of paper electrocardiographic printouts to digital electrocardiographic files. J Electrocardiol 2005;38:310–8.

38. Merri M, Benhorin J, Alberti M, et al. Electrocardiographic quantitation of ventricular repolarization. Circulation 1989;80:1301–8.

39. Laguna P, Thakor NV, Caminal P, et al. New algorithm for QT analysis in 24-hour Holter ECG: performance and applications. Med Biol Eng Comput 1990;28:67–73.

40. Malik M, Batchvarov VN. Measurement, interpretation and clinical potential of QT dispersion. J Am Coll Cardiol 2000;36:1749.

41. Elming H, Holm E, Jun L, et al. The prognostic value of the QT interval and QT interval dispersion in all-cause and cardiac mortality and morbidity in a population of Danish citizens. Eur Heart J 1999;19: 1391–400.

42. Ahnve S. Correction of the QT interval for heart rate: a review of different formulas and the use of Bazett's formula in myocardial infarction. Am Heart J 1985; 109:568–74.

43. De Bruyne MC, Hoes AW, Kors JA, et al. Prolonged QT interval predicts cardiac and all-cause mortality in the elderly. Eur Heart J 1999;20:278–84.

44. Malik M, Hnatkova K, Kowalski D, et al. QT/RR curvatures in healthy subjects: sex differences and covariates. Am J Physiol Heart Circ Physiol 2013; 305:H1798–806.

45. Lewek J, Ptaszynski P, Klingenheben T, et al. The clinical value of T-wave alternans derived from Holter monitoring. Europace 2016. http://dx.doi.org/10.1093/europace/euw292.

46. Baumert M, Porta A, Vos MA, et al. QT interval variability in body surface ECG: measurement, physiological basis, and clinical value: position statement and consensus guidance endorsed by the European Heart Rhythm Association jointly with the ESC Working Group on Cardiac Cellular Electrophysiology. Europace 2016;18:925–44.

47. Dobson CP, Kim A, Haigney M. QT variability index. Prog Cardiovasc Dis 2013;56:186–94.

48. Van Noord C, Eijgelsheim M, Stricker BHC. Drug- and non-drug-associated QT interval prolongation. Br J Clin Pharmacol 2010;70(1):16–23.

49. The Sicilian gambit. A new approach to the classification of antiarrhythmic drugs based on their actions on arrhythmogenic mechanisms. Task Force of the Working Group on Arrhythmias of the European Society of Cardiology. Circulation 1991;84: 1835–51.

50. Locati E, Schwartz PJ. Prognostic value of QT interval prolongation in post myocardial infarction patients. Eur Heart J 1986;7(Suppl A):393–8.

51. Rudehill A, Sundqvist K, Sylvén C. QT and QT-peak interval measurements. A methodological study in patients with subarachnoid haemorrhage compared to a reference group. Clin Physiol 1986;6:23.

52. Wahbi K, Algalarrondo V, Becane HM, et al. Brugada syndrome and abnormal splicing of SCN5A in myotonic dystrophy type 1. Arch Cardiovasc Dis 2013; 106:635–43.

53. Wilson FN, Macleod AG, Barker PS, et al. Determination of the significance of the areas of the ventricular deflections of the electrocardiogram. Am Heart J 1934;10:46.

54. Schwartz PJ, Priori SG, Locati EH, et al. Long QT syndrome patients with mutations on the SCN5A and HERG genes have differential responses to Na+ channel blockade and to increase in heart rate. Implications for gene-specific therapy. Circulation 1995;92:3381–6.

Moving?

Make sure your subscription moves with you!

To notify us of your new address, find your **Clinics Account Number** (located on your mailing label above your name), and contact customer service at:

Email: journalscustomerservice-usa@elsevier.com

800-654-2452 (subscribers in the U.S. & Canada)
314-447-8871 (subscribers outside of the U.S. & Canada)

Fax number: 314-447-8029

Elsevier Health Sciences Division
Subscription Customer Service
3251 Riverport Lane
Maryland Heights, MO 63043

*To ensure uninterrupted delivery of your subscription, please notify us at least 4 weeks in advance of move.

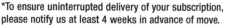

ELSEVIER

Moving?

Make sure your subscription moves with you!

To notify us of your new address, find your **Clinics Account Number** (located on your mailing label above your name), and contact customer service at:

Email: journalscustomerservice-usa@elsevier.com

800-654-2452 (subscribers in the U.S. & Canada)
314-447-8871 (subscribers outside of the U.S. & Canada)

Fax number: 314-447-8029

Elsevier Health Sciences Division
Subscription Customer Service
3251 Riverport Lane
Maryland Heights, MO 63043

Printed and bound by CPI Group (UK) Ltd, Croydon, CR0 4YY

03/10/2024

01040385-0007